Overcoming Common Problems

Living with a Heart Bypass

Dr Robert Povey, Dr Claire Hallas and Dr Rachel Povey

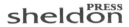

sheldon **PRESS**

First published in Great Britain in 2006

Sheldon Press
36 Causton Street
London SW1P 4ST

British Library Cataloguing-in-Publication Data
A catalogue for this book is available from the British Library

ISBN-13: 978-0-85969-918-1
ISBN-10: 0-85969-918-8

1 3 5 7 9 10 8 6 4 2

Typeset by Deltatype Limited, Birkenhead, Merseyside
Printed in Great Britain by Ashford Colour Press

Contents

Acknowledgements

We are most grateful to all those who consented to being interviewed as part of the background research for the book. The names and some details of people's case histories have been changed in order to protect anonymity, but all the histories are based on real-life studies of people who have undergone bypass operations and/or related medical investigations.

We are also indebted to the many people who gave so generously of their time in advising on certain issues or commenting on parts of the book. In particular we would like to thank Professor Peter Weissberg, Belinda Linen and Julia England at the British Heart Foundation; Elsa Griffiths, Royal Brompton and Harefield NHS Trust; Jane Thackwray, Mark Elliot and Ian Taylor, East Kent Cardiac Rehabilitation Team; Sarah Pullen, Gloucestershire Hospitals NHS Trust; Aly Chapman, Manchester Diabetes Centre; and Keith Jackson of the British Cardiac Patients' Association. We are also most grateful to Keith Lovet Watson for providing the humorous illustrations; and to the British Heart Foundation for permission to reproduce illustrations from Booklets 10 and 18 in their Heart Information Series.

Finally, we wish to say a special thank you to our 'other halves' – Lyn, Stef and Andy – for their invaluable support and encouragement during the writing of the book.

1

Life before a bypass: two case histories

The experience of those waiting for a heart bypass can be likened to the experience of people in a heavily congested town waiting for a bypass relief road! The road bypass will take much longer to arrange than a routine heart bypass operation, of course, but there are some interesting parallels. The long-suffering inhabitants of the gridlocked town may become resigned to the view that this is how life is going to be. They come to believe that the town's congested streets and poor traffic flow is unlikely to improve, and that they simply have to make the best of the situation.

Similarly, where people have perhaps suffered from the undiagnosed symptoms of heart disease for months or sometimes years, they may simply come to accept that their problems are an inevitable consequence of the stresses of modern life, or of the ageing process. They resign themselves to accepting their symptoms – the frequent bouts of what may feel like 'painful indigestion', or the tendency to 'get out of puff' when doing even minor physical activities – as something they just have to live with.

However, just as the problems inflicted on the town by the congested road links can be freed up by a bypass, so the symptoms experienced by people with coronary heart disease can be relieved by appropriate medical or surgical action. In coronary heart disease the main culprits that give rise to the person's symptoms are the furred-up, narrowed arteries supplying the heart; and fortunately, these can generally be modified, or bypassed with replacement blood vessels, so that the heart once again receives a sufficient supply of blood to enable it to work effectively. These blood vessels (the so-called coronary arteries) can become damaged in both men and women and in all age groups, for a variety of reasons which we will explore in Chapter 3.

The important point to remember, though, is that the problems produced by coronary heart disease can normally be relieved by changes to a person's lifestyle, by medication, or by surgical intervention such as heart bypass surgery. In the same way that the town-dwellers can start to look forward to a less congested town centre and a better quality of life following the building of a bypass relief road, so the person with coronary heart disease can look forward to life-enhancing changes once remedial steps have been

1

taken – and for many people (around 30,000 each year in the UK alone) this means heart bypass surgery. When a successful heart bypass has been carried out it will transform the blood flow through the cardiovascular system (the heart and its related blood vessels) and provide a welcome relief from the debilitating symptoms of heart disease.

The following case studies describe two very different experiences of life before a bypass. In both cases the underlying disease process – the narrowing of the coronary arteries – had almost certainly been developing for many years, but the heart problems only became clearly apparent when symptoms emerged that disturbed the individual's ability to perform everyday tasks. The case studies demonstrate the range of pre-bypass experiences, from David's slowly emerging but manageable symptoms, leading to an eventual bypass after several years of medical treatment, to Peter's sudden episodes of heart-related problems in which the symptoms were so severe and disabling that they resulted in an immediate hospital appointment and a heart bypass within weeks.

David

David is a single man in his early seventies. A retired university lecturer specializing in nineteenth-century literature, he had always enjoyed good health, apart from recurring headaches which he put down to pressure of work. He is a non-smoker, does not drink to excess, and had been used to taking regular brisk exercise, especially swimming and tennis. Like his mother, who died from a coronary in her eighties, David began to suffer one or two slight pains in his chest during his late fifties. Both he (and his mother before him) put these initial pains down to indigestion, although they turned out, in fact, to be angina.

The worst bout of these 'indigestion' pains occurred when David was 58. He was sitting up in bed one Saturday night reading when he suffered some strong pains across his chest which gradually got worse, eventually radiating down his left arm. He got up and fetched a medical dictionary and concluded that he might be suffering from a hiatus hernia. He poured himself a drink of milk and took a couple of antacid indigestion tablets and waited for the pain to subside. The next day the pains had more or less gone and he carried on with his usual Sunday activities, mowing the lawn and weeding the garden. But in the evening the pains returned and he decided to seek medical advice. His own doctor was on leave and he was seen by a locum GP who agreed that it was probably indigestion. He prescribed some slightly stronger antacid medicine. However, the pain continued, and as soon as his GP returned, David went back to see him. The doctor, suspecting angina, referred him for tests at the local hospital. He was given an ECG (electrocardiogram) test, which records the rhythm and electrical activity of the heart. The results revealed an abnormality, and David was referred to a consultant cardiologist (a doctor specializing in heart disease), who saw him a few weeks later. After further tests – several blood tests and an exercise or stress ECG (see pages 16–20) – the consultant confirmed that David was suffering from angina and that what he had thought was a severe bout of indigestion had been, in fact, a heart attack! But he had been lucky since it had not been a major heart attack and had not damaged his heart muscle too much.

David was given what he describes as 'a veritable medicine chest of prescriptions'. From being someone who had taken nothing more than the odd painkiller, David suddenly found himself on five lots of drugs. It was all a bit of a lesson in pharmacology! The 'medicine chest' included 50 mg atenolol per day, 20 mg isosorbide mononitrate twice a day, one 10 mg tablet of simvastatin to be taken once a day just before going to bed, and a 75 mg dispersible aspirin once a day. He was also given a glyceryl trinitrate spray to put under his tongue to help open up the blood vessels in an attack of angina. (See Chapter 5 for more on medication.)

David's GP explained the effects of the different drugs. He told David that the atenolol was a 'beta blocker' which would help to control the attacks of angina by regulating his heart rate and rhythm, so that there was less stress on the heart. Like the nitrate spray, but on a regular basis, the isosorbide mononitrate tablets would also help to keep angina at bay by dilating the blood vessels and allowing the blood to flow more freely. Taking simvastatin would reduce the total cholesterol level in his blood and help to prevent the arteries from becoming more furred up, and the aspirin would thin the blood to help prevent clotting.

David was seen once again by the consultant and then periodically by his GP over the next ten years, in which he was relatively free from angina.

During these ten years, David simply got on with his life, putting his intermittent symptoms down to 'the sort of problems you're bound to get with advancing age' as much as to the diagnosed heart problems. But the angina gradually started to get stronger and more frequent and David began to find that he suffered from quite strong pain at certain times during the day, for example, when he took his usual walk to the post-box in the evening after dinner, particularly on cold or windy nights. His GP decided that he ought to be seen again at the local hospital.

A new consultant, who also worked part-time at a London teaching hospital, was surprised that David had not been seen by a cardiologist during the intervening ten years. She remarked that 'You might be getting a bit older, but it's never a good idea to assume that all aches and pains are due to age!' After some preliminary tests, the consultant referred him immediately to a major teaching hospital for an angiogram (see the Glossary at the back of this book). The eventual outcome of David's tests was that he was put on the waiting list for a heart bypass operation.

Peter
Peter is a retired postman, married with grown-up children. His wife, Mary, works part-time at an Oxfam shop. They have been married for 45 years and have both enjoyed good health for most of their lives.

Peter has a family history of heart disease, his father having dropped dead from a heart attack at the age of 65. At the same age, just after he had retired from the Post Office, Peter suffered his first symptoms of what turned out to be heart disease. He was sitting in the car waiting for his wife to finish shopping in the supermarket when he began to feel faint and unwell. 'The world sort of closed in on me and I felt as if there just wasn't enough air . . . I was taken straight to the Accident and Emergency unit at the local hospital where they carried out tests . . . They kept me in for a week . . . When I was discharged I was put on 75 mg aspirin once a day and given a letter for my GP.'

A follow-up hospital consultation was arranged in three months. 'But before this came up I was back in hospital again, this time with a very rapid heart beat. I'd been swimming and it started when I was changing. After I got home my heart rate didn't calm down, so we sent for the GP and he called an ambulance . . . I was admitted to hospital and the consultant recommended that I should have an angiogram . . . I didn't even know what an angiogram was, but it was all very quick and efficient. After the angiogram, the doctor said, "It's a bit serious." I was in the corridor and I was a bit cold and shivering and he thought I was frightened. He said, "There's nothing to worry about." I told him, "I'm not shivering because I'm anxious – I'm shivering because I'm cold!" The consultant said I'd need five coronary artery bypasses and he wanted me to stay in and have them done straightaway. I went in for the angiogram on the Friday; I had the op on Monday and I was discharged on the following Sunday.'

Both David and Peter had successful bypass operations which removed their symptoms and allowed them to resume their normal everyday activities. But to explain how and why such heart problems arise, we look in Chapter 2 at the normal working of the cardiovascular system (the heart and its blood circulatory system), and in Chapter 3 at the factors contributing to cardiovascular malfunction.

2

A journey from the heart and back

We have already noted that the heart and its blood circulation system (the so-called cardiovascular system) controls the way in which blood is pumped by the heart around the body via the blood vessels. It's quite a journey, flowing through about 96,000 kilometres (60,000 miles) of vessels, from large arteries and veins to tiny blood vessels called capillaries. The journey would take you more than twice the way round the world!

The heart is a muscle, a bit bigger than the size of a fist, and it operates as a pump, with around 100,000 pumping operations (heart beats) every day. We feel the beats of the pump through an artery when we take our pulse rate. For example, if you place your index and middle finger over the underside of the opposite wrist, below the base of the thumb, you can feel the radial artery that supplies blood to the hand.

This life-maintaining pump constantly re-circulates about 5 litres (8 pints) of blood from the heart all round the body, through the arteries and then via smaller vessels (capillaries), before being collected from the capillaries by our veins. The branches of the veins join up to make bigger veins through which the dark, de-oxygenated blood circulates, passing through the kidneys and liver to drop off waste products, and then returning to the right side of the heart, as it relaxes in between contractions.

Figure 1 shows how blood circulates. The heart is made up of four chambers and has a one-way valve system so that the blood will only flow in one direction. The first two chambers (the right atrium and left atrium) act as collecting points for the blood before it enters the other two chambers (the right and left ventricles), which are the heart's pumping stations. In general, the arteries carry *oxygen-rich* blood away from the heart – but with one confusing exception. At the very beginning of the circulation cycle, after the returning blood reaches the right side of the heart, it is the pulmonary artery through which the *de-oxygenated* blood is pumped into the lungs where it rids itself of the carbon dioxide and picks up fresh oxygen; and it is the pulmonary *vein* that transports the oxygen-rich blood back to the heart.

After that confusing start, however, we're back to the arteries as the transport system for the oxygenated blood. The oxygen-rich bright-red blood is pumped from the left side of the heart, through the aorta around the body, dividing off into smaller and smaller blood vessels, until the

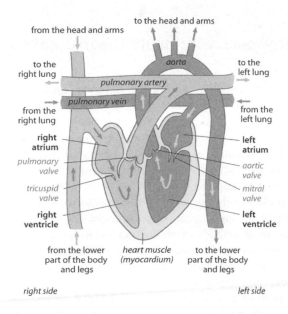

Figure 1 Normal heart function: how blood circulates

blood reaches every cell in the body, and then back from the capillaries, through the veins to the right side of the heart to start the whole process again, each cycle taking about 60 seconds.

The coronary arteries

Like any other muscle, the heart requires its own supply of blood in order to function properly, and this is supplied by the *coronary arteries* which lie on the outside of the heart muscle. (You can see the coronary arteries in Figure 2 on page 51, showing details of a procedure to open up a narrowed artery.)

Different coronary arteries provide blood to the different parts of the heart and its electrical system (the cells that generate electrical activity so that the heart will contract). This electrical system is the part of the mechanism of the heart that sometimes goes a bit haywire and requires a temporary 'electrical shock' input (or sometimes an artificial pacemaker fitted) to establish a regular heart beat again. The heart's natural pacemaker is located in the right atrium.

Problems with the functioning of the coronary arteries may lead to the need for a bypass operation and it is to these problems we now turn.

3

How and why heart disease develops

The factors contributing to the development of heart disease are many and varied. They range from genetic predisposition, to the effects of unhealthy lifestyles. People who inherit a set of genes linked to the development of heart disease (as in the case of familial hypercholesterolaemia, described on page 10) are predisposed to develop the disease; whereas people who take hardly any physical exercise, over-indulge in drink, eat a lot of foods high in saturated fat, and smoke, tend to *predispose themselves* to develop the disease.

In general, though, heart disease emerges as a result of the interaction of a number of these factors. Leading an unblemished lifestyle will not totally preclude the possibility of developing heart disease if your genes have given you a built-in vulnerability to the disease, but as we shall see later on in the book, following a healthy lifestyle helps to provide a valuable degree of protection from heart disease, or a platform on which to base a successful recovery from it. In card-playing terminology, the genes deal the cards but the environment determines how they are played!

Changes in the coronary arteries

Healthy blood vessels are flexible tubes, able to dilate easily in order to allow the blood to flow through them freely. In coronary heart disease, however, the blood vessels become furred up or narrowed (stenosis) and the blood flow becomes sluggish. This occurs as a result of the build-up of small fatty lumps called atheromas or atheromatic plaques (see the Glossary) to which certain types of cholesterol deposits (described below) make a major contribution. The condition in which the coronary arteries become narrowed in this way is called atherosclerosis.

When the coronary arteries become furred up, the blood and oxygen supply to the heart is reduced and this makes it much more difficult for the heart to do its work. It may be all right if you are taking it easy and not exerting yourself much, but when your heart requires more blood and oxygen – as, for example, when you begin to take more strenuous exercise or become emotionally stressed – then you may experience pains in the chest (*angina*). Sometimes these pains move to other parts of the body such as the left arm, as in

David's case (page 2), or the neck or jaw. If the build-up of the atheromatic plaques in the coronary arteries becomes too great, then the vessels may eventually become blocked and result in a cut-off in blood supply to the heart (called ischaemia). Such a blockage can happen suddenly, for example, when a blood clot forms on top of the atheroma. Then the artery can become blocked and this can lead to a heart attack.

Similarly, if the clot occurs in an artery supplying the brain, this can cause a cerebral thrombosis (stroke) and result in the death of a number of brain cells. This damage may affect speech, for example, or result in loss of movement or sensation in the arms, legs or other parts of the body, depending on which part of the brain is affected.

If the loss of blood supply to the brain is only temporary, this is known as a transient ischaemic attack (TIA), and such attacks tend to cause less severe damage than a fully blown stroke. Even with major strokes, however, there is a chance that, in time, other parts of the brain may gradually take over from the damaged areas so that some lost functions may be recovered.

In people requiring a bypass, there will have been some loss of blood supply to the heart. If the person has already suffered a heart attack, the muscular wall of the heart, called the myocardium, which is 'fed' by the coronary arteries, will have been starved of blood for a time. This is why you will find that a heart attack is often referred to as a myocardial infarction or MI (an 'infarction' denoting damage caused by lack of blood supply and 'myocardial' relating to the heart muscle). There's something quite snappy about using the term MI and many people seem to use this as a handy piece of medical jargon to describe their heart attack!

If the amount of heart muscle affected by the MI is relatively small, it may not prevent the heart from working effectively once the person has recovered from the initial symptoms (as in David's case described in Chapter 1, and Margaret's in Chapter 4); but it will be necessary to follow medical advice closely and to take relevant lifestyle measures to prevent a recurrence.

Some of the factors that help to trigger heart disease

Family history and genetic factors

There is a tendency for heart disease to run in families. Both David and Peter in Chapter 1 had a family history of heart problems, and heart disease that develops in a close relative under 50 can be regarded as a risk factor. Because families share a similar environment and often follow similar patterns in their eating, drinking and exercise habits, some of this 'familial' risk can be put down to lifestyle factors; but the combination of genes we inherit also has an important part to play.

This is especially the case in relation to a group of disorders known as familial hyperlipidaemias in which the pattern of gene clusters in individuals puts them at risk of developing coronary heart disease. One of the most severe forms of this disorder is called familial hypercholesterolaemia (FH), in which total cholesterol levels in the blood are raised to abnormal levels, as we will see in Margaret's case described in Chapter 4 (and see the section on cholesterol below). This disorder is also fully examined in *How to Keep Your Cholesterol in Check* by Robert Povey (Sheldon Press). Although we cannot at the moment control our genetic make-up, we are able to make clear choices in our lifestyles, and these can substantially modify the effects of our genetic inheritance.

The influence of genetic factors can also be seen in the regional variations in the incidence of heart disease. People of Celtic origin, for example, such as the Scots and Irish, have a high incidence of heart disease; whereas the Japanese have a low incidence, together with people born in Mediterranean countries such as France, Spain, Portugal, Italy and Greece. Similarly, Asians from the Indian subcontinent run a higher risk of developing diabetes than other nationalities, and this may be associated with a higher risk of heart disease.

However, genetic elements are only part of the equation, as we have already noted, and environmental factors have a major role to play in determining the level of risk experienced. So you find, for example, that when people move from the region where they were born and where there is a high incidence of heart disease (such as the USA) to a region with a lower incidence (e.g. one of the Mediterranean countries), then they tend to develop risk levels that are closer to their new country than to their country of origin. The most likely explanation is that people change their habits and adopt the healthier lifestyle and dietary approaches typical of people in their new country. We shall look in closer detail at the so-called Mediterranean Diet in Chapter 12.

Blood pressure (BP)

High blood pressure (hypertension) is a major contributor to heart disease, and, unfortunately, it often tends to remain a 'hidden' symptom. In fact, it is sometimes called the 'silent killer' because it can result in heart attacks and strokes without appearing to have caused any previous symptoms. The only way we can identify hypertension is by measuring our blood pressure. The measure used is called 'mm Hg' and this is based on the height in millimetres that a column of mercury reaches when blood pressure is taken.

In the traditional method, an inflatable cuff is placed around the upper arm and pumped up to apply pressure, then the air is slowly released until the pulse returns. A reading is taken at this point, denoting the maximum pressure in the artery when the heart contracts. This is called the systolic blood pressure (SBP). The cuff is then further deflated and a second, lower reading is taken (the diastolic blood pressure), representing the minimum pressure in the arteries in between beats, when the heart is at rest.

Readings persistently above 150/90 mm Hg are generally regarded as too high and the person is said to be suffering from high blood pressure (hypertension). The British Hypertension Society guidelines recommend that an optimal target for most people should be to try to keep below 140/85. For people with diabetes, the guidelines recommend even lower optimal targets – below 130/80.

Cholesterol

We have already seen that cholesterol deposits make a major contribution to the atheromatic plaques that lead to the narrowed arteries in heart disease. What we need to understand, however, is that not all forms of cholesterol are bad. In fact, this white waxy substance is an essential part of the membrane of each cell in our body; it helps to make bile which is used in digesting fatty foods, acts as an insulator for our nerves, and is involved in the production of hormones and Vitamin D. Most of our cholesterol is manufactured in the liver, utilizing substances that come from the fat in food – especially saturated fat, the sort obtained from animal sources as in butter, lard, cheese, fatty meat and full-cream milk. A small amount of cholesterol comes directly from foods such as meat and egg yolks. This is called *dietary cholesterol*, but it plays a relatively insignificant role in the development of heart-related problems.

The major culprit in causing problems for our coronary arteries is the cholesterol produced in the body via our intake of saturated fat – and, in particular, it is the type of cholesterol known as low density lipoprotein (LDL) that causes most of the damage.

Lipoproteins (or lipids) are the tiny packages that carry the cholesterol via the bloodstream to and from the cells. They differ in density and there are two main types, the low and high density lipoproteins (LDL and HDL). It may help to try to remember the difference in the following way: the **L**ow **D**ensity variety is **l**ess desirable, and the **H**igh **D**ensity variety is **h**ighly desirable.

- **LDL** ☹ People with high levels of LDL cholesterol in their blood are at increased risk of a build-up of cholesterol deposits which fur up the arteries and lead to coronary heart disease.
- **HDL** ☺ People with a high ratio of HDL cholesterol to total cholesterol in their blood have some protection from developing furred-up arteries, since HDL cholesterol seems to act like a scavenger, picking up excess cholesterol from the blood vessels and carrying it back to the liver to be reprocessed as bile.

These two types of cholesterol are affected by diet and exercise. We can lower LDL by reducing our intake of foods high in saturated fat, and we can help to increase HDL cholesterol by exercising more and by modifying our diet in certain ways (see Chapter 12).

We also discuss in Chapter 12 how our intake of certain foods and drink can help to control some other very low-density lipids that contain triglycerides, which are made in the liver or obtained from fat in the foods we eat. These are an important source of fuel for our bodies, but when the level of triglyceride in the blood is too high it can lead to blood clots and an increased risk of developing coronary heart disease. Excessive levels of triglyceride are also associated with diabetes and obesity, both of which are risk factors for heart disease.

The blood levels of the different lipids are measured in millimoles per litre of plasma (the fluid part of blood in which the white and red blood cells and other substances are suspended). In the USA they are measured in milligrams per decilitre. These measures are abbreviated to mmol/L and mg/dL, respectively. As broad general guidelines at the time of writing, for most people *without heart disease* medical experts tend to advise the following levels:

- Total cholesterol below 5.0 mmol/L (195 mg/dL)
- LDL below 3.0 mmol/L (115 mg/dL)
- HDL above 1.0 mmol/L (40 mg/dL)
- Triglyceride below 1.7 mmol/L (150 mg/dL)

However, people who already have heart disease, or who have had a bypass, are usually advised to apply more stringent targets. As one cardiac nurse puts it: 'We look for cholesterol scores preferably in the 3s for people who have had a bypass, but anyway less than 4 total, and less than 2 for LDL, and probably most cardiologists would say as low as it can go.'

Diabetes

In diabetes, the body's capacity to convert sugar from food we eat into energy is malfunctional, resulting in excess glucose in the blood. It's not entirely clear why diabetes should increase people's risk of developing atherosclerosis and heart disease. However, it is known that people with diabetes tend to have other risk factors associated with heart disease such as raised systolic blood pressure and triglyceride levels, together with low HDL cholesterol levels. This applies to people who develop diabetes when they are young (Type 1 diabetes) and require regular injections of insulin, as well as to people with Type 2 diabetes, which usually develops later in life (as in Stephen's case described in Chapter 5). Although in Stephen's case insulin injections were eventually necessary, Type 2 diabetes can often be treated by diet alone, or by medication and diet, without requiring such injections.

Obesity

Weight is one of the factors that we can usually modify by diet and exercise (see Chapters 11 and 12). Obesity has become an epidemic, and in a national audit in England, nearly two-thirds of men, and over half the women, were overweight or obese, as defined in the chart on page 82. It may be the factors linked to obesity, such as lack of exercise, high blood pressure and diabetes, that make it so strongly associated with heart disease. But whatever the mechanism, sensible weight (and waistline) control is certainly an important element in the prevention and treatment of heart disease, and those who have had a bypass operation should avoid becoming overweight or obese.

Lack of exercise

There is clear evidence from research studies, such as the British Regional Heart Study, that people who exercise regularly are much less likely than their inactive counterparts to have heart attacks and strokes. In this study, the risk of stroke was six times greater for inactive middle-aged men compared with those who regularly engaged in vigorous exercise, even when allowance was made for the links between an inactive lifestyle and other risk factors such as obesity and high blood pressure. The beneficial effects of exercise are most clearly documented in men, partly because the majority of large-scale studies examining the issue have used male participants, but regular brisk exercise undoubtedly has the effect of keeping the cardiovascular system of both men and women in good shape.

Exercise helps to lower our average blood pressure level (although blood pressure will, of course, rise during the actual period of exercise itself) and also increases levels of the 'good' HDL cholesterol and lowers triglycerides. So exercising contributes very effectively to the smooth and efficient working of the heart and blood vessels (see Chapter 11).

Smoking

Smoking is one of the most potent factors triggering the changes to the coronary arteries in heart disease, and it also carries a high risk of stroke and a number of cancers, including cancers of the lung, mouth, larynx and oesophagus. Smokers tend to have lower HDL and higher triglyceride levels than non-smokers. They also have higher levels of fibrinogen than non-smokers – and when the levels of fibrinogen are excessive, our blood becomes sticky and has a greater tendency to clot. This is bad news for the smoker's coronary arteries and leads to a higher risk of heart disease and stroke. So the advice for those having bypass surgery, both before and after the operation is, always, to give up smoking (see Chapter 11).

Stress

A certain amount of stress is valuable in helping us to function effectively, keeping us on our toes and enabling us to meet life's challenges. Our bodies prepare for dealing with situations calling for 'fight or flight' reactions by producing more of the hormones adrenaline and noradrenaline, and these in turn put up our heart rate and blood pressure, raise total cholesterol, lower the 'good' HDL cholesterol and increase the tendency of the blood to clot.

For short-term emergency measures this is fine and the body sometimes needs to react in this way – but if we live our lives in a constant state of high arousal, this can have physical repercussions, and this is where stress can start to have detrimental effects on heart-health. In particular, people who exhibit certain types of behavioural traits such as aggression, competitiveness, anger and hostility tend to have an increased risk of developing heart problems; and these feelings can often do most 'internal' damage when they remain pent-up and simmering rather than outwardly expressed.

We offer advice on coping with stress in Chapter 14.

Gender

Men tend to be about three times as likely to develop heart disease as women. Until the menopause, women seem to be protected by the female hormone, oestrogen, but after the menopause they become more susceptible to developing the disease; and by the time people reach their mid-eighties, men and women have about an equal risk of having a heart attack. With bypass operations, taking all age groups into account, women generally account for less than a third of the total number of people having the operation, but they also tend to have smaller arteries than men, and this can sometimes make bypass surgery more intricate, as in Margaret's case, which is described on pages 20–3.

In the next chapter we look at how doctors decide when to recommend bypass surgery.

4
How doctors decide who needs a bypass

We have already seen in the two case studies presented so far that there can be many twists and turns in the route leading to a bypass operation, which, depending on the severity of symptoms, may be carried out within weeks, or delayed for years. During the intervening period medication will usually have been tried, together with lifestyle and dietary changes, until these are no longer working adequately and a bypass becomes essential.

The stage at which a bypass is carried out also depends to some extent on the individual assessments of cardiologists and surgeons, and on the hospital facilities available. However, the basic criteria will be the state of the cardiovascular system in general and the coronary arteries in particular, together with the severity of the symptoms produced – and these will be assessed using a number of different tests. Some of the tests may present temporary discomfort, as in the prick of a needle or having to be attached to a portable blood pressure monitor for 24 hours; but they don't, in general, pose any more problems than having something like a standard chest X-ray, for example, which may also form part of the preliminary pre-bypass test procedures.

Blood pressure, cholesterol and other routine tests

Your doctors will usually routinely check for problems with high blood pressure (hypertension) and abnormal cholesterol levels (dyslipidaemia). Dyslipidaemia means 'problems or difficulties with lipids' and covers a wider range of abnormalities (such as the important condition of *low* HDL cholesterol levels) than 'hyperlipidaemia', which only refers to *raised* lipid levels.

Your doctor will also usually carry out other blood tests to check on things like glucose levels, to identify whether there are any problems related to diabetes; and you might have blood tests to check the functioning, for example, of the liver and kidneys. Your doctor may ask you to fast for 12–14 hours before a blood test, if you are having your triglyceride levels or LDL cholesterol levels checked, for example, since these are affected by intake of food and drink. Some doctors may check the level of other substances in the

16

blood which have been shown to have relevance to coronary heart disease, such as homocysteine (low levels of which can be remedied by an increased intake of folic acid, found in green leafy vegetables and yeast extract); and a blood test for the level of your thyroid hormones may also be requested, since an underactive or overactive thyroid gland can be implicated in heart problems.

The electrocardiogram (ECG)

An ECG provides much more detailed information about the rhythm and electrical activity of your heart than does a stethoscope. The nurse will put several small sticky patches (electrodes) on your chest and limbs. These electrodes are connected to the electrocardiogram which records the electrical signals produced by each heart beat on a moving roll of paper. The test usually takes around five minutes, and can detect whether you have any significant problems with your heart rhythm; it can also sometimes indicate whether you have had a heart attack (MI) at some time (as in Margaret's case described later).

Sometimes doctors will carry out an ambulatory ECG (also called Holter monitoring), just as they can also arrange for an ambulatory ('walking') blood pressure check. With a blood pressure monitor, the person wears the usual cuff around the arm and it inflates and deflates, usually at 20-minute intervals, taking the person's blood pressure over a 24-hour period. For an ambulatory ECG, four electrode leads are fixed to the person's chest and linked to a small recording device (like a personal stereo) that is strapped to a belt round the waist. The person then carries on as normal for the 24-hour period, and indicates by pressing one of the buttons on the recorder if and when any worrying episode occurs (e.g. an angina attack).

Exercise or stress ECG

If the doctor feels it would be helpful to test your heart under more strenuous conditions, then an exercise or stress ECG might be arranged. You will be rigged up to the usual ECG monitoring device with electrodes on the chest, and a blood pressure cuff will be attached, so that blood pressure can also be monitored during the test, along with the heart rate and heart rhythm. You are then asked to walk on a treadmill, which will gradually increase in speed and incline. The heart is monitored constantly and any problems are noted. There may be evidence of abnormal heart rhythms, for example, or certain changes in the ECG tracing may indicate that the heart muscle is not getting enough oxygen-rich blood during exercise.

The doctor or technician will indicate when to stop (or you may ask to stop), and this will depend upon the nature of the readings on the monitor or the severity of any symptoms you are experiencing. In cases where the coronary arteries are severely blocked, for example, as in Margaret's case described below, the test may last only a very short time before it is brought to a halt. The results are usually quite helpful in determining the severity of the heart problems.

Echocardiogram

As the name suggests, this test involves the use of high-pitched echoes (beyond the range of human hearing) to build up a picture of the heart, using the ultrasound scanning method familiar to many pregnant women and also to people like Stephen (see Chapter 5) whose gallstones were discovered by a scan.

A lubricating jelly is spread on the chest to ensure satisfactory contact with the probe, which is then moved around so that a good picture of the heart is built up on the video screen from the echoes reflected through the machine. It is particularly useful in identifying problems with the heart valves, and was used to identify Margaret's pulmonary embolism (see end of this chapter).

Radionuclide tests

Sometimes the cardiologist will recommend a radionuclide scan (also known as an isotope or a thallium scan), which can check for a number of heart-related problems. When doctors are checking for coronary artery disease, a radionuclide test may be used before undertaking any more invasive techniques, such as an angiogram (see below). Often two tests are performed, one at rest and the second after exercise, and then the two scans are compared. The test indicates which areas of the heart appear to have inadequate blood flow – either because of narrowing of the arteries, or a previous MI.

For the scan taken at rest, a small quantity of a radioactive 'tracer' substance (isotope) is given intravenously and a couple of hours later, when the tracer has circulated sufficiently, the scan will be performed. The scan takes no more than half an hour. The person lies down and a large scanner is positioned over the chest so that it can provide images of the tracer, from different angles, as it passes around the heart. The scan taken after exercise is the same, except that after the tracer has been injected, the person is asked to exercise on a treadmill or exercise bike. If he or she cannot exercise sufficiently, a drug may sometimes be used which makes the heart pump harder and faster. Then the second scan is carried out.

Oddly enough, between the injection and the scan, the person is sometimes asked to eat the sort of foods, high in saturated fat, that they have been trying to keep to a limited intake – like chocolate bars or full-cream milk or cheese sandwiches! Some radiographers consider that because high-fat foods get the liver and gall bladder working hard, this will help to prevent the isotopes from being 'soaked up' by these organs, allowing more to reach the target organ, the heart – and so the images of the heart are likely to be better. For some people this gives the radionuclide scan an attractive bonus: 'I rather enjoyed having these tests because I don't normally eat chocolate bars . . . It was like being in heaven – eating chocolate bars as a 'reward' for doing the test, and without feeling guilty!'

Other scanning devices

Other scanning devices are occasionally used and include Positron Emission Tomography (PET), Magnetic Resonance Imaging (MRI) and Computed Axial Tomography (CAT) scans. They involve lying in a small 'tunnel' in a machine that produces images of various parts of the body. PET and CAT scanners are particularly valuable in detecting certain tumours, and MRI scanners are used frequently in neurological investigations. These devices can also provide information about the functioning of the heart, but are probably less frequently used in heart investigations than the scanners discussed earlier.

Coronary angiogram (or cardiac catheterization)

Often called the 'gold standard' test for coronary artery disease, this is carried out on a 'day patient' basis, before a decision is made to perform coronary angioplasty or bypass surgery. This is basically an X-ray test in which pictures are taken of the coronary arteries, but unlike standard X-rays which are taken from outside the body, it involves inserting a small tube called a catheter (about the width of a pencil lead) into a vein or artery, usually in the groin but sometimes in the arm. This is why it is sometimes described as an 'invasive' procedure. But although it might feel a little uncomfortable, it is painless and relatively straightforward. The site where the catheter is inserted is anaesthetized. The catheter is then guided with the aid of X-ray screening along the blood vessels until it reaches the coronary arteries, when a contrast dye (visible on X-rays) is injected into the arteries through the catheter, so that detailed pictures can be obtained.

You can sometimes follow the procedure on the video screen. One person found it 'interesting'; another 'watched the TV screen with anticipation but, being warm and comfortable, promptly went to sleep!' Other people prefer not to watch: 'I didn't particularly worry about it. I thought, "They know what they're doing" . . . I just left them to it!'

When the dye is injected you may feel a slight 'hot flush' for a couple of seconds, and some people experience slight angina pain, or fleeting palpitations, but there is usually little discomfort otherwise: 'I found that the most uncomfortable part was the prickly sensation in my groin afterwards, where I had shaved myself in preparation for the angiogram!' When the catheter is removed, the doctor or nurse will apply pressure to the groin for about ten minutes, or a plug (angioseal) will be applied to stop the bleeding. A slight bruise may develop at the site of the puncture after the test, but this disappears in a few days.

On the basis of the type of tests described in this chapter, your doctors will decide whether you need any treatment. Sometimes, like David in Chapter 1, people can manage for a time on medication; in certain cases (like Margaret's case below), a coronary angioplasty is required (see Glossary); and in others (as with Peter in Chapter 1), an immediate heart bypass will be performed.

In the next chapter we discuss the types of medicine used to control coronary heart disease before and after surgical intervention.

Margaret
Margaret is now in her mid-fifties. She used to work as a playgroup helper, but stopped work in her late thirties when she married Bill, a retired insurance salesman. A non-smoker, she had always eaten a healthy diet, was not overweight and took plenty of exercise.

Margaret went through the menopause early, and put down her feelings of fatigue at that time to menopausal symptoms. But these feelings of tiredness persisted and she asked her GP for his advice. He found that her blood pressure was a bit on the high side, but he didn't feel that this was anything to worry about. He encouraged her to try to avoid too much stress and to take plenty of exercise.

Over the next few years she carried on, still feeling very tired but without any other particularly concerning symptoms, until she visited her GP about a large yellow lump that had developed on her elbow, like a wart to begin with, which was gradually getting bigger. Her doctor passed her on to a specialist in skin disorders, who identified the yellow lump as a xanthoma, caused when there is excess cholesterol in the body – and a blood test did indeed confirm that Margaret had a very high total blood cholesterol level (14.9 mmol/L). The GP also asked about her relatives and discovered that there was an uncle and a brother who had died of heart disease at a young age. Margaret knew that her brother's cholesterol level had been very high, and both he and her uncle had diabetes. The GP explained that this suggested that Margaret's problems were caused by the inherited disorder called familial hypercholesterolaemia (FH), in which very high levels of cholesterol and xanthoma are classic symptoms.

The GP also discovered that Margaret's blood pressure was worryingly high (195/100) and prescribed medication for both her raised cholesterol and her hypertension. She was put on 40 mg atorvastatin to lower her cholesterol, and for her blood pressure she was given 10 mg amlodipine, a calcium antagonist (see Chapter 5). The doctor warned her to take things easy because she was at risk of having a heart attack; and told her that if at any time she started to feel unwell again he would refer her to a heart specialist.

However, she remained reasonably well for a couple of years, apart from the all-pervasive feeling of fatigue. Her xanthoma gradually disappeared, as her cholesterol level reduced, and she felt she might be getting things under control – until she began to experience some new symptoms.

When she was out walking, her breathing would sometimes become very heavy and she would start to get a tight chest. She went back to see the GP who diagnosed angina and gave her a nitrate spray to help to relax the arteries and relieve the pain. He also put her on 40 mg isosorbide mononitrate, which has the same effect as the spray but is more long-lasting, and he prescribed 25 mg of atenolol, a beta blocker to help to lower her blood pressure and also keep her angina at bay. She carried on for a few more months but the symptoms, though a little better, were still troubling her, and her GP finally referred her to a cardiologist.

Margaret was still very under the weather when she went to the hospital for her appointment, at which the cardiologist gave her a number of tests, including a resting ECG and a stress ECG. She had been given a standard, resting ECG some time before, and this had shown up some irregularities, but the test this time indicated that she had also suffered a slight heart attack at some point. Her doctor thought this was likely to have occurred during her recent episode of severe chest pain, but he wanted to assess her on a stress ECG test in order to see how serious her problems had become. Margaret found that even with only a slight increase in the gradient and speed while walking on the treadmill, she was unable to continue with the test because the angina pain was too strong; and the cardiologist recommended that Margaret should have an immediate angiogram. He also counselled her to take it very easy until he had been able to perform the angiogram. She went into hospital as a day patient for this test.

The images revealed that there were several narrowed arteries and one that was almost blocked. In the cardiologist's view this needed coronary angioplasty and this was duly performed together with the insertion of a special 'drug-eluting stent', a small piece of metal mesh coated with a drug to hold the semi-blocked artery open (see Chapter 8).

During the next six months she felt better and was able to walk without much discomfort, but her condition then gradually started to deteriorate again. 'I was getting breathless . . . and I had another chest pain . . . this was really severe. So my husband rang the ambulance and they took me to hospital.' The doctors found from their various investigations, including an ECG, a radionuclide scan, and an echocardiogram, that it wasn't a heart attack (or MI) – on this occasion it was a pulmonary embolism. The doctors explained that one blood vessel in the lungs had become blocked as a result of a blood clot, and it was fortunate that she had come into hospital for treatment so quickly since this can often be fatal. After this, Margaret was prescribed warfarin, a blood-thinning drug, for six months and put on the waiting list for a heart bypass. She was also referred to cardiac rehabilitation classes in the meantime, so that her condition could be monitored.

Unfortunately her condition did not improve. When she was at the rehab classes she couldn't really complete her exercises because she got so breathless. She was advised not to push herself, and to stop doing the exercises if she was in any discomfort. She went back to see her GP, who decided that she looked so poorly she should be admitted to hospital as an emergency. Another angiogram was performed and they found this time that the artery that had the stent was now completely blocked. They decided to do a triple bypass straightaway.

The operation took quite a long time because Margaret's arteries were small, but it was very successful and the surgeon was pleased with her recovery. As far as drugs were concerned, Margaret was kept on her cholesterol-lowering medicine (40 mg atorvastatin), and also prescribed 2.5 mg ramipril (an ACE inhibitor), in addition to atenolol (now at 50 mg per day) in order to keep her blood pressure under better control. To keep her blood thin, she was also put on 75 mg clopidogrel instead of aspirin – which tended to upset her stomach. (When aspirin had been prescribed previously in the hospital, she was given a dose of 30 mg lansoprazole each day alongside it to treat her sensitive stomach – and she was pleased now, with clopidogrel, that she only needed to take one tablet instead of two.) Her cholesterol post-bypass was 4.8 and blood pressure 137/76.

When Margaret went to see the surgeon after the bypass he told her that her arteries were very small and that he had to work 'twice as hard for his money' that day! But he was very reassuring: 'Let's put it this way,' he said, 'it's like an MOT for the car. You have to be careful, but at least you have about 21 years of good life ahead of you.' She was chuffed at this vote of confidence, and was keen to pass on the benefit of her experience to other people in a similar position. Her advice to anyone who is being encouraged to have a bypass is: 'Go for it!' She says you only need to think about what life was like before the bypass – 'Just climbing up the stairs made me feel so unwell but now I feel a new person!'

5

Medication used in coronary heart disease

A whole variety of medicines are used to treat coronary heart disease, alongside lifestyle measures such as diet and exercise. As we have already seen in our case studies, the types of medication prescribed depend upon the nature of the problems, and the preferences of the medical team. However, there are sufficient common features to enable us to summarize the most usual forms of drug treatment.

As far as side effects are concerned, we will mention some of the most common ones, but on the whole it's probably best to avoid looking too assiduously for side effects because you can tend to become a little preoccupied with the search. As one person put it: 'The trouble is, you read about all the side effects on the leaflet, and you think, "Yes, I get that, and that . . . and that . . ." and you end up thinking all your aches and pains come from your tablets! . . . I've decided it's best just to note down anything that's *really* unusual . . . and then I tell the doctor about it.'

Your doctor will often want to carry out blood tests after (sometimes before *and* after) you start taking particular medications, to check that the drugs don't have any adverse effects on organs like the kidneys and liver. The types of medication described in this book represent the drugs most commonly prescribed by doctors at the time of writing.

Medication for high blood pressure (anti-hypertensive drugs)

Since high blood pressure (hypertension) is one of the most common risk factors for coronary heart disease, drugs to treat this are among the most frequently prescribed for those who are either at the pre- or post-bypass stage. Some anti-hypertension drugs, such as atenolol, for example, also provide effective treatment against angina (and may be classified as both anti-hypertensive and anti-anginal prescriptions). We will mention the dual classification of such drugs as we examine the main categories of anti-hypertensive drugs, the first of which includes a range of 'blockers'.

Beta blockers

Beta blockers have both anti-hypertensive and anti-anginal effects and so they are frequently prescribed for potential bypass candidates. They work by blocking the receptors in our cells that help to facilitate the actions of the hormone adrenaline. This hormone exerts its chemical effects on our bodies, and especially on the heart, when we are under stress or excited. The adrenaline rush makes our heart work harder and faster, and increases our heart rate and blood pressure. Beta blockers help to slow down the heart rate, lower blood pressure and reduce the heart's demand for oxygen. They also have the effect of controlling angina and protecting the heart muscle from undue exertion following a heart attack.

Because beta blockers slow down the heart rate, people sometimes find that they make them feel a bit tired, or cold (especially in the hands and feet), and they may exacerbate asthma. But on the whole they are well tolerated and, if you do find you don't get on with one particular beta blocker, there are quite a few for your doctor to choose from! It is important not to stop taking beta blockers suddenly since this may result in a worsening of symptoms. Some of the most widely used beta blockers are: antenolol, bisoprolol, metoprolol, propranolol and sotalol, but this is by no means an exhaustive list.

ACE inhibitors

ACE stands for 'Angiotensin Converting Enzyme', and drugs that inhibit this enzyme help to prevent the conversion of angiotensin I into angiotensin II, which is a 'neurohormone' and has the effect of constricting the arteries. The technical name for something that constricts the blood vessels is 'vasoconstrictor', and angiotensin II is a powerful vasoconstrictor that has the effect of forcing up the blood pressure. When the arteries are constricted it is much more difficult for the blood to flow through them, and thus higher blood pressure is required to force the blood through. By blocking this 'constriction' process, the medication helps to keep the blood vessels dilated (that's why these drugs are sometimes called 'vasodilators') and so it helps to *reduce* blood pressure and makes it easier for the heart to pump blood around the body. The drugs also help remove excess fluid from the body.

In addition to their value in the treatment of hypertension, ACE inhibitors help the heart muscle to function after a heart attack and, like the A2 antagonists described below, are useful in helping to reduce the risk of kidney disorders in people with Type 2 diabetes. These drugs are also valuable in cases of *heart failure* – which doesn't mean that the heart has packed up altogether, but that it is not pumping as well as it should be. Commonly prescribed ACE inhibitors are captopril, enalapril, lisinopril, perindopril and ramipril. One of the annoying side effects can be a persistent dry cough.

Angiotensin II antagonists – also called ARBs (Angiotensin II Receptor Blockers)

These are very similar to the ACE inhibitors, but they act by blocking angiotensin II (or A2) receptors *directly*. It's a bit like a game of musical chairs where the receptors are the chairs and there is a competition to sit in them. The substance (angiotensin II in this instance) has to sit in these chairs to function properly. What the angiotensin II blockers do is to sit in the 'receptor' chairs before the substance gets there, thus preventing it being able to operate effectively.

One beneficial effect of this difference in operation between ARBs and ACE inhibitors is that people don't tend to get the dry cough with ARBs. These drugs have also been shown to be particularly beneficial for people with blood glucose problems and they might even help to reduce the chances of developing Type 2 diabetes (see page 13). Commonly used ARBs are candesartan, eprosartan, irbesartan, losartan, telmisartan and valsartan.

Calcium antagonists

These drugs may be used in both anti-hypertensive or anti-anginal treatment. A certain supply of calcium is essential to ensure that the heart muscle works effectively, but a reduction can have beneficial effects on both the heart and on the arteries. Calcium antagonists (sometimes called calcium channel blockers) reduce the amount of calcium available and the overall effect of this is to reduce the heart's contractions slightly and relax the blood vessels so that they widen and make it easier for the heart to pump blood around the body.

There are a variety of calcium antagonists which have different effects on the body and are used for different heart conditions, e.g. diltiazem and verapamil tend to reduce the usual level of heart rate occurring on exercise; whereas nifedipine (see Stephen's case below) and amlodipine (Margaret's case in Chapter 4), prescribed in these two instances as anti-hypertensives, are primarily vasodilators (i.e. they relax or dilate the blood vessels).

As with beta blockers, you are advised not to stop taking calcium antagonists suddenly since this may result in a worsening of the symptoms of angina. With the primarily vasodilator versions of these drugs, 'flushing' (in which the person gets sudden 'flushes' of blood, showing, for example, in the reddening of the face or neck) may be a nuisance as a side effect.

Diuretics (water tablets)

Diuretics, or water tablets, work on the kidneys, the organs that sift waste products and excess water from the blood and excrete the waste as urine. The drugs increase the amount of water and salt eliminated from our bodies through the urine, leading to a reduction in the volume of blood and hence to a lowering of blood pressure. Some diuretics, especially loop diuretics (see below) are also used to treat heart failure in which the reduction in the heart's capacity to pump blood around the body results in oedema (the accumulation of fluid in the tissues). So someone with heart failure may find that they have swollen ankles or legs, or that they become breathless (when the fluid accumulates in the lungs). Diuretics can help such conditions.

There are three main types of diuretic – thiazides, loop diuretics and potassium sparing diuretics.

Thiazides

These are frequently used to control high blood pressure, and one of the most commonly prescribed drugs is bendroflumethiazide. Usually taken in the morning, the drugs act within a couple of hours and last for 12 to 24 hours.

One drawback with thiazides is that they can lead to a loss of potassium, and so your doctor will order a blood test to check on this. There are plenty of foods rich in potassium (e.g. apricots, bananas, raisins), but for some people a potassium supplement may need to be prescribed.

Thiazides can also have a detrimental effect on blood glucose levels, and so this is another aspect your doctor will check.

Loop diuretics

These are very fast-acting drugs. They are called 'loop' diuretics because they work on part of the kidney called the 'loop of Henle'. When taken orally, loop diuretics work within an hour and last for between four and six hours, producing an increased urine output. They are usually taken once a day in the morning, but sometimes people will be asked to take them twice a day. It is usually recommended that the second dose is taken in the afternoon rather than late in the evening, to save having to get up in the night. Like thiazides, these drugs can lead to a loss of potassium. Two of the most commonly prescribed loop diuretics are frusemide and bumetaride.

Potassium sparing diuretics

These diuretics help the body to retain potassium and are, therefore, often combined with thiazides and loop diuretics. Commonly used drugs are spironolactone and amiloride.

Medication for dyslipidaemia

The most commonly used drugs for the control of lipid abnormalities, such as raised total cholesterol, are statins. The main drugs you are likely to come across are atorvastatin, fluvastatin, pravastatin, rosuvastatin and simvastatin, sometimes in conjunction with other drugs (e.g. ezetimibe plus simvastatin). They act on the liver to reduce its production of cholesterol, so total cholesterol is lowered; and they will also help to lower triglyceride levels and to *raise* levels of the desirable HDL cholesterol. By reducing total cholesterol, and especially the 'less desirable' LDL cholesterol, the statins help to slow down the development of atherosclerosis. Indeed, these drugs have been so successful in helping to prevent and treat heart disease, that a small dose (10 mg) of simvastatin is now available as an 'over-the-counter' medicine which can be purchased without a prescription by people at moderate risk of developing coronary heart disease.

For people with existing heart disease, or for those who are post-bypass, these drugs are normally part of the medication regime and can have a dramatic effect on lipid levels alongside dietary measures. Margaret's total cholesterol level was eventually reduced from an extremely high 14.9 mmol/L to 4.8 mmol/L on a dose of 40 mg atorvastatin per day (see page 23). Statins are taken at night because this is the time the liver produces most of its cholesterol. They are generally well tolerated, with few side effects, although you should inform your doctor if you experience any unexplained muscular pain that you have not experienced before taking them. It should also be noted that people taking some of the statin drugs (atorvastatin and simvastatin, in particular) are advised not to drink grapefruit juice since this interferes with the processing of the drugs in the liver and can result in higher than desired statin levels in the blood. You will be advised to complement these drugs with exercise and diet (see Chapters 11 and 12).

Medication to prevent or disperse blood clots

Anti-platelets

These drugs, along with other blood-thinning preparations, are used to prevent the formation of clots in the blood vessels. They act by reducing the action of platelets (cells in the blood that help in the clotting process). The most commonly used anti-platelet is aspirin. Most of those with heart conditions, at both the pre- and post-bypass stages, will be taking a regular low dose of aspirin, usually 75 mg per day. It helps prevent heart attacks in people with coronary heart disease, and also reduces the risk of stroke caused by a cerebral thrombosis (a blood clot in the brain). It will also be prescribed as a 'maintenance dose' after a heart attack or bypass. Aspirin may sometimes cause irritation to the stomach, but this is not usually a problem in small doses (and, if necessary, medication can be prescribed to counteract the problem). Sometimes a drug called clopidogrel is used instead of aspirin for those who find aspirin difficult to tolerate (see Margaret's case in Chapter 4). It may also be used for short periods along with aspirin, for example, following an episode of unstable angina (see page 32) or as a precaution in coronary angioplasty with stenting to reduce the risk of blood clotting after the procedure (see Robin's case, described on pages 53–4).

Clot busters

In situations where a clot needs to be dispersed very rapidly, as for example with a clot that has formed in a coronary artery leading to a heart attack, the person may be given a clot buster drug. The most common are probably streptokinase, anistreplase, tissue Plasminogen Activator (tPA) or reteplase, which are given intravenously, either by injection or drip. Technically, these types of drug are called thrombolytics or fibrinolytics. In the case of streptokinase and anistreplase, once you have been given the drugs you are not able to have them again because the body produces antibodies against them; so you will be given a card to say when you were given them.

To stop more clots from forming after a heart attack or thrombosis, people are also sometimes given drugs known as anticoagulants, the most common of which are heparin and warfarin. Heparin is given by injection and works more or less instantly, whereas warfarin is given orally and takes a couple of days or so to become fully effective, and may be prescribed to be taken for a few weeks or months, as in Margaret's case following a pulmonary embolism (see Chapter 4).

Medication for the relief of angina

Glyceril trinitrate

Look in the pocket or handbag of someone suffering from angina and you are likely to find a small spray known as a glyceril trinitrate (or GTN) spray. This, or a small tablet which has the same effect, is sprayed (or placed, in the case of a tablet) under the tongue and a small amount of a nitrate is dispensed which acts as a vasodilator (dilating the blood vessels), thus improving the supply of oxygen and blood to the heart muscle. The effect is quite rapid and the nitrate begins to work as soon as it is absorbed (usually less than a minute). So whenever you feel the angina pain, it's best to stop, sit down if possible, use your spray or tablet, and rest until the pain subsides.

You can also use the spray before you start on a walk, or any activity you think might bring on your angina. Some people find that the GTN spray brings on a bit of a headache, but the dilemma between relieving strong angina pain or having a brief headache is one that usually resolves itself in favour of the headache!

When more sustained nitrate absorption is considered necessary, to prevent rather than alleviate angina attacks, it can be used in patches on the skin, or in tablets such as isosorbide mononitrate. Any side effects such as flushing, headache or dizziness (opening the blood vessels will tend to lower blood pressure and this may cause you to feel a bit woozy occasionally) are the same as for the GTN spray, but these do tend to diminish with time.

Potassium channel activator

Another anti-anginal drug that has a nitrate-like action and has similar side effects is nicorandil – technically called a potassium channel activator. It acts as a vasodilator and is used for the prevention and treatment of angina.

These are the types of drugs used for those with coronary heart disease, and combinations of these drugs and others will be prescribed both before and after a bypass operation. The British Heart Foundation produces an excellent series of booklets on all aspects of heart disease and its treatment, including one called *Medicines for Your Heart*. Details of all their booklets can be found on their website (see page 120).

Stephen's case (below) illustrates many of the issues we have examined in the previous chapters. It shows how many factors interact to trigger the changes in the cardiovascular system which can lead to heart disease and eventual bypass surgery. It also illustrates how, with the aid of skilled medical and surgical intervention, and by people themselves taking determined steps to improve their diet and lifestyle, the problems can be tackled very successfully.

Stephen

Stephen is 58 and a retired social worker, married with three grown-up children. His wife, Deborah, is also a social worker. Stephen retired early, at 50, because of stress at work, which was exacerbated by ill health brought on by undiagnosed gallstones and diabetes. He had suffered from pains in his abdomen for some time before an ultrasound scan identified that he had gallstones; and his diabetes was only diagnosed during a routine blood test when he was in hospital having his gall bladder removed! In retrospect, he realized that his excessive thirst and tiredness (which he had put down to stress) were both related to his untreated diabetes.

Stephen had been treated for raised blood pressure and high cholesterol for some years. He tended to get overweight, and he had been given advice on diet and exercise. He was also advised to stop smoking, and was prescribed medication – 30 mg nifedipine, a drug known as a calcium antagonist (see page 26), for hypertension, and 40 mg simvastatin to bring down his cholesterol. These measures worked well. His blood pressure was reduced from 180/100 to an average of about 130/80 and his cholesterol from 8 mmol/L to around 4 mmol/L. He tried to keep fit by swimming and walking, and eating a healthy diet. He was not aware that he had any other medical problems until he was diagnosed in quick succession with gallstones and diabetes. His health had not been good and the diagnosis came as something of a relief since it made sense of the symptoms he had been experiencing and he now knew the problems were treatable.

He was given dietary advice at the hospital when his diabetes was diagnosed. Stephen didn't need insulin at this stage, although he had to start taking it later on, a few months before he went in for his bypass. For the time being he was treated by diet and tablets (500 mg metformin three times a day) for his Type 2 diabetes. This drug is one of the so-called oral hypoglycaemic drugs – taken orally and designed to bring down the amount of glucose in the blood to normal levels.

He was also advised (again) to give up smoking. He'd smoked ever since he was a teenager and regularly smoked about 30 cigarettes a day. 'It was agony, giving up; but I knew I had to for the sake of my health. I'd tried before when my GP discovered my blood pressure and cholesterol problems. I cut down a bit, but I slipped back into my old habits.' However, after Stephen's cholycystectomy (removal of the gall bladder) and the diagnosis of diabetes he thought, 'Now I've got to do it.' 'So I stuck at it – used patches and other aids. But in the end it's just mind over matter, really. I thought, "I'm not going to let it beat me." This habit was dictating my life, and I'm not going to let it do that.'

Stephen's heart problems didn't become apparent until after his early retirement, and then they were only intermittent. He suffered from pains in his chest on exertion, particularly when gardening. He didn't do anything much about these symptoms to begin with, thinking they might be connected to his diabetes.

But his chest pains gradually got worse and eventually angina was diagnosed, for which Stephen's GP prescribed 25 mg of the beta blocker, atenolol. When Stephen found he was getting the pains at rest, however, the GP became worried that this could be unstable angina, which he viewed with rather more concern than the stable angina he had been treating. Stable angina occurs more or less predictably on exertion and so is relatively easy to control, whereas unstable angina is less predictable, occurring at rest as well as with exercise.

The GP arranged for Stephen to have an 'ambulatory ECG' for which he was wired up to a portable ECG machine for 24 hours. This revealed sufficient irregularities for the GP to send Stephen for a stress ECG test at the hospital. (These ECG tests are described in Chapter 4.) The results confirmed that he had some distinct heart problems for which he was referred to a consultant cardiologist who arranged for him to have an angiogram (see Chapter 4).

'They decided to use a vein in my wrist rather than the groin to insert the probe. I'd shaved my groin and it was all ready down there, but they decided on the wrist, which pleased me because they said it tends to heal a bit quicker there . . . It shocked me when the doctor came round to see me afterwards and said I'd got three blocked arteries and I needed surgery. I suppose I hadn't really thought I was going to need it . . . I felt a bit hot and sticky then! . . . I was a bit happier when another doctor suggested later on that they could try me on medication for a bit to see if this would sort it out . . . They put up my dose of atenolol from 25 mg to 50 mg, kept me on the 30 mg nifedipine and 75 mg aspirin, and added a small dose of isosorbide mononitrate, to improve the blood flow, as they put it.'

However, after a few weeks on this medication it was decided Stephen should see the consultant heart surgeon again. As he entered the consulting room, Stephen was greeted by the words 'I'm surprised you're still here . . . haven't you had a heart attack yet?' It was uttered in a jocular fashion, but it wasn't quite the greeting Stephen had expected, and he began to feel a bit faint! According to Deborah, Stephen's wife, this news had quite a marked effect on Stephen's behaviour afterwards. 'He was afraid to walk too far with the dog in case something happened to him, whereas he'd never thought about it before . . . It knocked his confidence. I went grey with worry too. If he wasn't back at the usual time I started to get really anxious.'

Stephen was given all the preliminary details about having a bypass and told that they would try to fit him in as soon as possible. A very short time afterwards Stephen attended a follow-up Cardiology Outpatients' clinic. The pains in his chest and neck had become much worse and instead of leaving for home after his consultation he was admitted straight into the Cardiac Care Unit: 'Although this was a bit of a shock, it was also a relief – the thought that I was in the right place and something was going to be done.'

The operation was carried out successfully and his post-operative care in hospital was generally straightforward. He did have some very vivid dreams as a result of the drugs used during the operation (such drug-induced effects can also sometimes include brief hallucinatory experiences), and he found it difficult for a short time to distinguish which events were real and which ones were imagined.

But the only disturbing event of any *physical* significance during this period was the occasion on which his heart went out of rhythm: 'I was quite unconcerned and unaware of any problems until they told me! Apparently it was caused by a low potassium level.' In hospital they controlled this by drugs, but Stephen was also told that his potassium levels could be kept up 'by eating a couple of bananas a day' (see also page 84 on potassium in foods).

When he left hospital the beta blockers were stopped, but he was kept on simvastatin to control his cholesterol levels, insulin and metformin for his diabetes, and 75 mg aspirin to help prevent blood clots. He was also prescribed DF 118 painkillers. Later, ramipril 10 mg, an ACE inhibitor (see page 25), was added to control his hypertension. Stephen's blood pressure is now regularly around a healthy 130/80.

After he got home, Stephen had one or two temporary 'memory lapses' which he thought might be related to the operation: 'They mention in the leaflets that your memory can sometimes be affected, and I wondered whether I might be able to get away without paying my bills because of loss of memory! . . . But I didn't notice anything really that bad.'

He attended the rehab class organized by the cardiac rehab team: 'I thought it was excellent, and I'm carrying on after the eight weeks . . . you have to pay a bit then . . . but it's very helpful . . . I'd advise anyone needing a bypass to go and have it done. It'll improve your lifestyle enormously . . . and having the operation is not as daunting as you imagine beforehand.'

6

Diagnosis and the waiting
period before surgery

This chapter focuses first on dealing with the *diagnosis* of heart disease, and then on the *waiting period* between being advised by your cardiologist that you need to have a heart bypass and being admitted to hospital for surgery.

Dealing with the diagnosis

There are some common phases in the adjustments people make to any stressful situation, and these apply to those recently diagnosed with heart disease. These may include shock and disbelief, or denial, which generally occur after experiencing severe symptoms or after getting the diagnosis; and these reactions may be followed by a period of 'grieving'.

Shock and disbelief may last a couple of weeks or so, and this can be psychologically protective, allowing you time to distance yourself emotionally from the new situation for a while, until you have managed to come to terms with the reality. This involves taking on board the nature of your cardiac problems and finding ways of adapting to them. The bypass surgery itself, and the rehabilitation programmes afterwards, play a major part in helping you to adjust, both physically and emotionally – and by learning how to self-manage your physical health effectively, you will find that this also has an enormously beneficial impact on your psychological well-being.

Try not to worry about time scales – putting pressure on yourself to come to terms with the diagnosis, treatment and potential outcome of your cardiac problems too quickly is unrealistic. Try to take one step at a time along the road to treatment and recovery. This will put less pressure on you and help to give you time to think through the information you are being given, and the decisions you are required to make.

Grieving

You may feel as if you are grieving – grieving for your lost health, for your life as you knew it, or for your plans now put on hold.

These emotions are a normal part of accepting the cardiac problems. But remember that this grieving is just a phase – and in most heart bypass cases, something of a premature emotion. Because one huge advantage of bypass surgery is that it often enables people to get back to their old lifestyles just as before, but *better*, because their new life is now free from the debilitating symptoms of heart disease, such as painful angina. In Robert's case, for example, his concern that he would be unable to ski again was banished within a year of his bypass (see page 76). For others, moving on from the grieving phase may involve a re-evaluation of their lifestyles and a search for new and different challenges in the future.

Coping with the waiting period and preparing for your bypass

There will usually be one or two preliminary visits to the hospital for pre-surgery assessments and pre-admission advice, and then it's a question of waiting until you reach the top of the waiting list and you receive a letter confirming the date for admission. The time period will vary depending on the hospital's waiting list times, the surgeon's waiting list times, your individual needs and the urgency for cardiac surgery.

Waiting for a major event to happen in our lives is often stressful even when that event is a happy one, such as a wedding in the family; but waiting for a bypass can present additional problems because of the nature of the cardiac problems involved. Some people are able to carry on with most of the usual physical activities in their everyday lives without undue concern, whereas others are severely limited in the activities they can perform, and may become anxious and stressed doing things that involve only minimal exertion. David, for example, was able to carry on mowing his lawn and going on his usual walks despite angina, whereas his friend felt very anxious about doing any physical activity and was unable to 'walk the width between two lamp posts' (see page 59).

Anticipatory anxiety

The waiting period for bypass surgery is frequently described as the most stressful part of the whole process. People face a great deal of uncertainty and often feel that they are not in control of events – not knowing how long they will have to wait for the operation or whether their heart condition is likely to worsen while they are waiting for the bypass. This is when people tend to feel more anxious than at any other time. This state of mind is sometimes described as *anticipatory anxiety* and is characterized by the posing of 'What if?' questions.

Robert (see Chapter 10) describes such anticipatory anxiety very clearly. He recalls that 'the idea of having to wait several weeks or even months before having my heart bypass worried me. I was very concerned that my condition would deteriorate before the surgeons could get at me! I wasn't particularly bothered about the operation itself. If it had to be done, then let's get it done. It was the thought, "What if I die before I get to the top of the waiting list?" – that's the scary bit. They told me that I was in urgent need of an operation, but they didn't really reassure me that I'd get it in time. Probably they couldn't because of "waiting list" problems.'

This anticipatory anxiety is also graphically expressed by Sheila (see Chapter 14). She describes the waiting period as 'horrible . . . the worst time of my life. I just went completely numb. Perhaps it was also because my mother had just died and perhaps it was the thought that for so many hours I wasn't going to be in control of my body.'

But both Robert and Sheila coped with their anxieties effectively in their different ways. Robert focused on routine work matters while keeping as fit as possible so he would make a good recovery after the op. Sheila concentrated on arranging family matters and post-bypass care, and even planned her funeral to minimize potential confusion and distress for her family. 'I told my son, who is 34, that he would find my birth certificate, pension book and funeral arrangements in the top drawer in my bedroom. I don't know who looked worse, him or me! It's funny . . . you start tying up loose ends . . . it's almost as if you're not sure whether you're going to die or come back.'

Different types of coping strategy are discussed later on in this chapter, but first we examine the role that emotional factors play in our attempts to come to terms with the planned bypass operation.

The importance of emotional factors in preparing for a bypass

So far, the main emphasis has been on the physical symptoms associated with cardiac disease. In this chapter, though, we focus on the psychological or emotional aspects of living with cardiovascular symptoms, and particularly on the management of thoughts and emotions while waiting for bypass surgery.

It's important to acknowledge your thoughts, feelings and

emotions about the forthcoming bypass so that you can deal with them effectively. It can be a worrying time, raising many questions and concerns, and can bring about strong emotions that you do not routinely experience. The result of such emotions can sometimes be quite distressing. People who are advising you (especially the healthcare professionals like doctors and nurses) will reassure you that it is normal to feel anxious, low in mood or lacking in confidence; and it's true that it is a normal response to feel like this *initially* when you are trying to come to terms with your diagnosis. However, it is *not* normal to continue to feel this way over any length of time. Feelings that are overwhelming, or interfere with your ability to carry out everyday activities while waiting for surgery, do not have to be experienced or 'put up with', and you should seek help from your GP if you feel unable to cope. We also discuss a number of coping strategies later on in this chapter.

Strong emotions such as anger, anxiety and frustration may have a negative impact not only on your capacity to cope with challenging situations, but also on your ability to take in information, and make appropriate decisions about your state of health. In fact, the persistence of such strong emotions over a long period of time can ultimately change the way your cardiovascular system functions. For example, there is clear research evidence showing that people who experience persistently high levels of anxiety are more prone to raised levels of heart rate and blood pressure than less anxious individuals; and these physiological changes can have adverse effects both on symptoms before bypass surgery and on the speed of post-surgical recovery. So it's important to try to keep things in perspective.

If you are finding waiting for the op difficult, try not to bottle up your feelings. Talk things over with a friend or with your practice or cardiac nurse, and make sure your GP keeps a close eye on your physical symptoms. If it's necessary to get you in for a bypass earlier rather than later, remember that it may be possible to move urgent cases rapidly up the waiting list (see Stephen's case, page 33).

Variation in people's responses to cardiac problems

Cardiac problems are not invariably the same from person to person, and people's experiences vary according to the nature of their symptoms and the treatment they receive. Similarly, when coming to terms with such problems there isn't just one right way of dealing with them, as we've seen with the different ways in which Robert and Sheila coped with their pre-op anxieties.

Sometimes, of course, the pattern of cardiac problems and coping strategies *will* follow a similar pattern to those of other people you know or have heard about. Sheila's symptoms, for example, replicated her father's experiences in some respects (see page 106). But there is no reason why you *should* react in a similar way to other people. The word 'should' initiates a set of expectations in your mind and then this benchmark of expectations acts as a 'judge' in relation to your *actual* behaviour. This may, of course, be rewarding if the judgement is that you have coped well with a difficult situation in a manner that is in line with the benchmark expectations.

However, it can also be unrewarding, and you may even feel as if you are being 'punished' if you consider that you have let yourself down because you haven't lived up to the benchmark expectations. So while it is important, and often very helpful, to take note of other people's experiences, it's also important to remember that people differ in the way that symptoms affect them and the way in which they react to their symptoms.

How emotions may affect your everyday life during the waiting period

There may be a variety of different emotions and issues to consider. Although maintaining your physical health and fitness for surgery will be a priority, it is also important to maximize the quality of other areas of your life. Remember that although you are waiting for surgery and may feel 'in limbo', this is still an important part of your life and there will be events during this period that you will look back on with pleasure in future years. Your active and enjoyable personal life may have to be curtailed in certain respects, but it doesn't have to stop just because you are waiting for a bypass. Being aware of how emotional (and physical) aspects of your life impact on your routine is important, of course, but the best way of dealing with this is by acknowledging them and finding ways of accommodating them. Tackling such issues before surgery will also give you confidence and awareness of possible difficulties *after* surgery.

The emotional upheaval during this period may well have adverse effects on your ability to cope with routine tasks. Problems considered relatively normal include:

- Reduced concentration and attention (e.g. when reading, watching TV, performing tasks, hobbies).
- Short-term memory problems (e.g. because of 'things on my mind').

- Relationships (e.g. having more of a 'short fuse' with other people).
- Sleeping difficulties (delayed onset of sleep or early morning waking due to worry).
- Changes in (or loss of) appetite (may be affected by low mood).
- Lack of motivation or interest in hobbies or daily routines.

Negative and positive feelings – the 'rollercoaster' ride of emotions

Most people waiting for a bypass op experience a combination of both negative and positive feelings. This 'rollercoaster' ride of emotions can fluctuate, just as it does for people without heart conditions – for example, coping with changes in health, hot or cold weather, dealing with everyday events such as the arrival of unexpected bills or the eruption of family disputes. People react to challenging situations in different ways, depending on their underlying personality characteristics and coping styles. Some of the feelings (both negative and positive) that people most frequently report while waiting are summarized below:

Negative feelings

- Anxiety and increased worry (with or without feelings of panic).
- Reduced confidence and/or frustration with the physical limitations imposed by the symptoms of heart disease.
- Low mood from time to time ('fed up', 'What's the point?').
- Anger ('Why me?').
- Fear (of surgery and/or symptoms).

Positive feelings

- Hope (about the future, improved health, reduction in symptoms).
- Elation, happiness, optimism (being given a 'second chance' and the likelihood of improved lifestyle after treatment).
- Motivation (to get better, to do more physically, to 'get on with life').
- Gratitude for the support and care of family and friends.

It can be helpful to keep a record of the times during the day, or the particular situations, that make you feel most happy or positive (and also most unhappy and negative). You can then try to find ways of increasing the number of 'positive' situations you encounter (and, similarly, reducing the 'negative' ones) and so help to lift your mood. This is sometimes called 'proactively targeting positive experiences'!

While most people manage to cope with the waiting period without getting too downhearted, the ups and downs (especially the downs) can have a draining effect if they go on for too long. However, by monitoring your own particular rollercoaster circuit you can understand the ways in which you respond to challenging or stressful situations. Generally, we need to adjust slowly to new situations and events in our lives, and remember that we all have good days and we all have bad days – this is normal irrespective of whether we have health problems or not.

Strategies for coping while waiting for your bypass

Previous examples in this book have highlighted how sudden, new or unexpected cardiac symptoms can act as triggers for people to change the way they conduct their routine and daily activities. This can feel unsettling or strange at first. Stephen felt uneasy about walking his dog too far from home in case he had a heart attack (see page 33). Drawing on positive styles of coping, however, will help to maintain emotional stability and relieve some of these unsettling feelings. For Stephen, taking the practical step of making sure he had his nitrate spray with him gave him the reassurance he needed. So it's useful to identify coping approaches that will be most helpful in dealing with your symptoms while you are waiting, and in enhancing your recovery from surgery afterwards. Equally it's useful to know which approaches are best to avoid.

Ways of coping that are generally unhelpful and best to avoid

- Denying that any action is needed ('sticking one's head in the sand') – in other words, prolonging for too long the initial disbelief and denial.
- Avoiding dealing with problems which then become too large to ignore and may turn into a crisis.
- Using substances such as alcohol, smoking or drugs to 'blot out' problems or divert away from them.
- Resisting and avoiding change (e.g. lifestyle changes, including modifications to exercise and diet) (see Chapters 11 and 12).

Ways of coping that are generally helpful

- *Adopting a determined stance not to let the 'illness take over'*

View the waiting period as a challenge and opportunity rather than a threat. Keep a sense of your identity, who you are, your likes and

41

dislikes, your goals, hobbies and plans. Keep up some of your leisure activities even if they are much reduced compared with the time before your symptoms appeared.

- *Taking a positive and proactive perspective on issues*

Try to see 'the other side of the coin' rather than just accepting the gloomy side and, like Robert (page 74), keep ahead of the game by anticipating problems and introducing ways of managing or solving them at an early stage.

- *Planning and preparing activities carefully*

Prioritize needs and base your activities around your choices. Pacing yourself will maximize the length and frequency of activities you can undertake. This will also reduce the impact of fatigue and physical limitations on your quality of life. Don't avoid activities unless medically advised to do so. This can undermine your confidence and make it more difficult for you to return to them after your bypass. Also, make sure you reward yourself for your achievements during this period.

- *Keeping as fit as possible and taking precautions to avoid infections*

Making sure your body is as fit as possible is a good preparation both for your surgery and for your recovery afterwards. Try to keep to a healthy weight (see Chapter 11) since excess weight can increase the risk of complications during surgery. It's also important to avoid infections, including teeth and gum infections (so a pre-op dental check-up is sensible), in order to prevent surgery having to be postponed.

- *Engaging in 'pre-hab' activities supervised by a cardiac rehab team*

Some people with heart disease, like Margaret (page 22), are fortunate enough to be referred to a cardiac rehabilitation unit *before* their bypass, so they can build up their pre-surgery fitness. As a cardiac nurse explains: 'Even the higher-risk bypass patients do much better post-surgically if they have exercised on a rehabilitation programme beforehand, called "pre-hab".' This emphasizes the importance of exercising before your bypass.

● *Using the support of friends and family*

Talking with a supportive person about your worries can help you to resolve them. As Margaret puts it: 'Being told I was to have a bypass did worry me ... but I thought, "Well, if it does you good, let it be ..." I've got a good friend, a good listener, and I talk to her when I can't get rid of my anxieties.' You can take along members of your family, or friends, with you to your consultations. It's often difficult for one person to take in everything that is said during a consultation, and an extra person will help you to remember the main points made by the doctor or other health professionals. It's also extremely valuable to have a supportive person to discuss things with after the consultation.

● *Using distraction techniques if particularly anxious*

Keep busy. Playing music, writing letters or cards, sending text messages on a mobile phone, reading books or magazines and doing active tasks that involve some problem-solving (e.g. crosswords or Sudoku puzzles, or fixing something that's broken) will help to distract you from your anxieties.

● *Talking through your concerns with health professionals and others*

If you are struggling emotionally, do not accept feeling unable to cope. Request professional help via your GP or talk with the staff or fellow 'patients' if you are having 'pre-hab'. Margaret found both staff and others in the joint pre-hab/rehab group very reassuring and positive: 'Several people had already had a bypass, and told me not to worry. At one session, an ex-patient talked to the group. He said, "Look at me, I'm well. I had it done ten years ago." It's all in the mind ... If you're positive about it, it's better.'

● *Recognizing the need to organize personal affairs*

Try to deal with any unresolved issues prior to surgery – for example, make a will, deal with any financial concerns, sort out detailed arrangements with your family, as Sheila did. Robert strongly advises people 'to try to sort out any paper work about sick pay and claims to Social Security before you go in for the op, especially if you're self-employed. Because it's so difficult to

43

concentrate on that sort of thing when you come out. I think it would be a good idea, when you're filling in all the preliminary assessment forms at the hospital, if someone went through with you details about sick pay before you go in for the operation . . . They tell you to avoid stress – but when you've got all these worries to deal with, it's impossible!'

- *Clarifying your expectations of bypass surgery*

Clarifying your expectations of surgery and checking how realistic these are will form an important part of the waiting period. This is where your post-operative rehabilitation goals begin to be shaped. These expectations will differ from person to person. For example, someone who has had painful arthritis for several years and has already experienced difficulty in walking before the onset of angina, would not expect to walk without arthritic pain after the bypass, but should expect relief from the pain of angina. In contrast, another person whose heart has the same pumping capacity and whose arteries have suffered from the same degree of atherosclerosis, but does not suffer from arthritis, will realistically expect to be without the pain of angina and also to be more active.

- *Making practical preparations for your immediate admission to hospital*

We discuss these in the next chapter.

Thinking ahead to the time you will spend in hospital is sometimes uncomfortable because of natural anxiety about undergoing cardiac surgery. But you are also likely to feel positive anticipation that through the surgical and rehabilitation processes you will obtain relief from the debilitating symptoms of heart disease and learn how to self-manage your cardiac problems effectively. The next chapter describes the start of this journey to a new life, free from these debilitating symptoms – the admission to hospital.

7

Going into hospital

When you receive the date for your hospital admission, you are likely
to feel relief that the waiting is over, and also some apprehension
about what is to come. Unless you have been in hospital before, it will
feel like something of an adventure into the unknown, but for most it
turns out to be a very welcome adventure which transforms their lives.
Margaret describes her own transformation: 'It's amazing the things
that inhibit you before . . . like being unable to walk to the shops and
back . . . You don't have these problems afterwards . . . it's trans-
formed my life.' As for Sheila, she thinks, 'It's the best thing you'll
ever have done . . . I've been given a second chance!'

At the end of this chapter we list ten questions we hope will remind
you of some important issues to consider before you embark on this
'adventure'. Some of these questions may already have been answered
during your pre-admission meetings with doctors or other health
professionals. Sheila found her pre-admission sessions to be very
helpful and informative: 'You can take a member of the family, and
they talk about everything – going in before, and aftercare . . . my
daughter came with me both to the angiogram and when I went in for
the op, and my granddaughter came to the pre-bypass interviews at
which the health professionals told me everything I wanted to know.'

Robert was also very satisfied with his pre-admission advice: 'I
was given a folder providing an induction into the procedure. It took
you through everything quite helpfully. A sort of reference guide – it
told me how the operation worked, what to expect. Very clear . . . A
nice nurse introduced herself to me and said I'd be on her ward.'

But not everyone finds that pre-admission discussions answer *all*
their questions. In fact, however much information you are given,
you are still likely to find you will have loads more questions you
want to ask later. An experienced cardiac nurse explains: 'A lot of
the pre-admission advice is given on one day at the hospital, and it's
difficult to take everything in – it's only when people get home that
they realize they still have a lot of questions unanswered. If they
have been on a waiting list for six months, they will have generated
a lot of questions, and the short time they are in the hospital for their
pre-assessments often doesn't give them long enough to have them
answered. Fortunately, people often just want very practical advice
before the bypass – what does the partner need to do, what transport

is available, where to stay, how do you get home, and all these are usually answered satisfactorily before admission.'

Your GP and his or her team, or the cardiac rehab staff, will be able to handle questions that crop up after discharge.

Before admission, you are likely to have received information in leaflet or booklet form from the hospital, and this will be supplemented by further information you will receive from your rehab team *after* you have had your bypass. Some hospitals have a detailed information booklet that will prepare people for what to expect when they come into hospital *and* during their period of recovery at home. You may also be given a copy of one of the excellent British Heart Foundation information booklets, such as *Having Heart Surgery*. (These can be obtained from the British Heart Foundation: see page 120.)

Contents of information sheets given to those having bypass ops before they are admitted to hospital

The exact nature of the information varies from hospital to hospital, but you are likely to be given the sort of information described below.

Information about admission procedures

This will include a preliminary letter detailing the date for admission, advice about what medication you will need to stop taking and when to stop taking it, and details about any important telephone contacts you may need at the hospital in order to finalize arrangements or clarify points. You will also be given a list of 'What to bring into hospital' (like nightwear/slippers/dressing-gown, toothbrush/toothpaste, glasses, reading material, medicines you are taking) and 'What not to bring' (e.g. large amounts of money or valuables!).

Advice will be given to you about travelling arrangements to and from hospital, and the importance of having someone to accompany you and carry your bags when you make the journey home. The leaflets may also discuss issues such as taking sick leave from employment and the need to sort out details about claiming any benefits to which you are entitled while you are off work.

You may be given details about pre-surgery procedures, including the need to sign a form of consent for surgery, and the physical preparations once you are in hospital, such as removing hair from parts of the body that will be involved in surgery, e.g. chest, legs, groin; showering with an antibacterial solution the night before the op; and not eating or drinking anything for six hours or so before the op. The sequence of events on the actual day of surgery may also be described, e.g. no food or drink before your op, pre-op shower, 'pre-med' (preliminary medication before you go to surgery, usually in the form of a tablet, to make you feel drowsy), being taken to the operating theatre and given an anaesthetic drug in a vein to send you off to sleep; and then being taken to the recovery unit, and later back to the ward.

You may be given information about recovery on the ward – how best to help your body make a swift and full recovery from the operation, including diet and exercise. Your exercise programme will be supervised by physiotherapists and nurses, and the information sheet may mention a target exercise that the staff would like to see you carry out before you leave hospital, such as walking up and down stairs.

Some advice may also be contained about what to do when you return home (e.g. what sort of exercise to take, and how much) – or this may be given in a separate 'discharge' leaflet (as described in Chapter 9). It may also explain details about your post-surgery medication – in particular, that you will be given a sufficient supply of tablets to tide you over the initial couple of weeks or so after you get home. You will usually be given the names and phone numbers of important contacts such as your cardiac nurse, and given details about a cardiac rehabilitation programme and any follow-up appointments with the cardiac surgeon's team.

Information from other people with similar experiences

You will no doubt hear stories from others who have had a heart bypass and such stories are often very reassuring – although they can also cause some anxiety if the person has had a negative experience. But we have already seen how beneficial such contact can be, with Margaret's description of the support she received before her bypass (page 42), while David watched video clips of people talking about their successful bypass operations.

Sheila has some interesting comments: 'An ex-bypass patient who did voluntary work at the hospital came round to talk around the fourth day after my op . . . I feel personally that perhaps someone should do that *before* you have the op. Because I think if someone like this came to see you while you were waiting to have your op, that would have been really good.' [This is arranged in some hospitals; and the British Cardiac Patients' Association – page 120

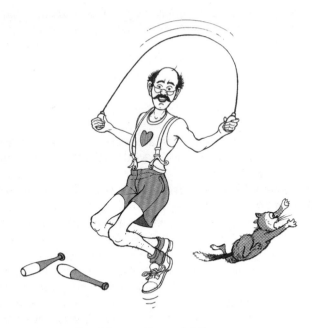

Looking quite sprightly . . .

– also has a list of members willing to share their experiences with pre- or post-bypass patients.] 'Just before I left I was waiting for my daughter, and this husband and wife came and you could see in their faces, she was frightened for him and he was frightened. And I said to her, "I'm going home. I've had the op. I'm well." She said to her husband, "That lady's had the op" . . . And it made such a difference to them. If they did that, it could help a lot of people.'

Stephen also describes the benefit he gained before his op from talking to someone who had already had the same op: 'There was an elderly gentleman in his eighties looking quite sprightly, doing his exercises and already looking forward to driving down to Spain in his motor caravan. He told me that when he came round from the operation he didn't even realize that he'd had the op! I thought it can't be all that bad then! He was a real encouragement. And according to one of the registrars, he wasn't the oldest patient they'd had. They'd carried out a successful bypass on a man who was 92 years old!'

Ten questions to help with your transition to hospital

Now here are the ten questions we think may help you to clarify any final queries you have, set out as a checklist you can tick off to reassure yourself that you are as well prepared as you can be.

1 Do I need any extra information now about bypass surgery to reassure me, or to help me think through my recovery?
2 Am I clear about how long I am expected to stay in hospital and what I need to bring with me?
3 Am I clear about what types of procedures/treatments I'm likely to have after the surgery?
4 Do I know the visiting arrangements at the hospital, and have I discussed these with the people who I'd most like to have around while I'm in hospital? (See also Question 6.)
5 Have I thought about who is aware of my stay in hospital and would be able to deal with my personal affairs if necessary?
6 Have I thought about how I will be feeling emotionally after surgery and if I am likely to want/need support from a friend or family member?
7 Do I need to arrange any care, support or assistance for my family, pets or dependants while I'm in hospital?
8 Do I need to discuss any further information, or make additional arrangements with my workplace or with benefit agencies?
9 Am I clear about how well I am likely to be able to cope with various aspects of home life when I return home from hospital (e.g. personal care, domestic jobs, shopping, cleaning, cooking, childcare)?
10 Will I need to rearrange some aspects of my home life, or require extra support in the short term while I'm recovering?

You will have been given a number of contact names and telephone numbers during your pre-admission discussions with the hospital, and if you are still unclear about anything in the above list of questions, you should be able to find answers from them, or from your GP or practice/cardiac nurse, or from this book.

8
Coronary angioplasty and bypass surgery techniques

In this chapter we look first at what happens when you have coronary angioplasty, as in Margaret's case (Chapter 4), and then at how coronary bypass surgery is carried out.

Coronary angioplasty

Coronary angioplasty was introduced in 1977, and now some 45,000 angioplasties are performed in the UK each year and about a million a year in the USA. Most of these are 'planned' angioplasties after angiograms, but sometimes the procedure may be carried out as an emergency procedure for a condition called 'acute coronary syndrome'. This occurs when the doctors aren't sure whether the person is having a heart attack or is suffering from unstable angina (which comes on with lower and lower levels of exercise and even when the person is at rest). In such situations, doctors may decide to perform the procedure immediately.

Normally, however, the doctors will have identified a narrowed coronary artery from the initial angiogram and the angioplasty will be carried out in order to widen this artery to improve the blood flow to the heart. The procedure is broadly the same as that adopted for the angiogram (see page 19), using X-ray screening to position the catheter, but instead of a plain catheter, this procedure uses a balloon-tipped catheter. This is the basic angioplasty equipment which allows for the small balloon to be inflated when it reaches the narrowed part of the artery so that it effectively 'squashes back' the atheroma plaques in the artery wall.

At one time this 'balloon angioplasty' was the main technique used, but this is now usually supplemented by the use of a stent, a tiny tube made of stainless steel mesh also carried in the catheter (see Figures 2 and 3).

The guide wire of the catheter goes just beyond the narrowed part of the artery (see Figure 2) and the balloon and stent are positioned within the narrowed section. Then the balloon is inflated and the stent expands to hold the artery open, as can be seen in Figure 3.

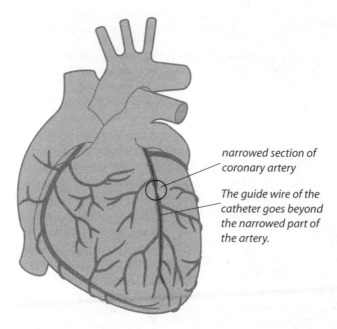

narrowed section of coronary artery

The guide wire of the catheter goes beyond the narrowed part of the artery.

Figure 2 Coronary angioplasty with stent: positioning the catheter

Finally, the balloon is deflated and removed together with the catheter, leaving the stent in position to keep the artery open, and allowing the blood to flow freely through it once again. The use of stents has provided a major improvement in the angioplasty procedure and reduces the chances of the artery becoming blocked again (restenosis). There are two types of stent: the most usual kind is the standard bare metal stent, but there is also a variety called a drug-eluting stent which is now increasingly preferred, especially for people with small arteries, like Margaret. The drug-eluting stent is coated with a special drug to help reduce the risk of the artery becoming blocked again.

If you have angioplasty with a stent the doctors will give you anti-platelet drugs (see page 29) – for example, clopidogrel plus aspirin to be taken both before and after the procedure. These will help to prevent clots and to reduce the chances of the artery becoming blocked again. The doctors may also give other anti-platelet drugs intravenously (called glycoproteins IIb/IIIa inhibitors) during the procedure. As in Margaret's case, some people may also be advised to take an anticoagulant drug such as warfarin for a few months afterwards.

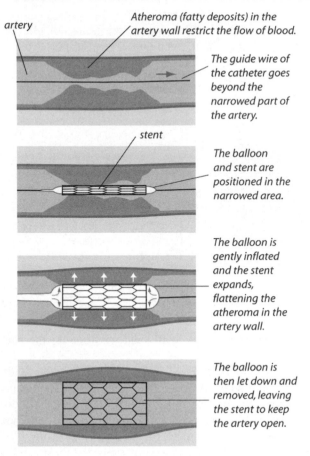

artery

Atheroma (fatty deposits) in the artery wall restrict the flow of blood.

The guide wire of the catheter goes beyond the narrowed part of the artery.

stent

The balloon and stent are positioned in the narrowed area.

The balloon is gently inflated and the stent expands, flattening the atheroma in the artery wall.

The balloon is then let down and removed, leaving the stent to keep the artery open.

Figure 3 Coronary angioplasty with stent: how the stent is inserted

In the majority of cases, angioplasty with a stent (or stents) is a successful procedure and can be carried out either on a day-patient basis or with an overnight stay. You will need to take things a bit easy for a few days, but most people are usually able to resume their normal activities, including driving, after a week. You may also be given the opportunity of joining a cardiac rehabilitation programme afterwards. If the angioplasty doesn't sort out the problem, a heart bypass may become necessary (and in a very few complicated cases, where the artery becomes totally blocked during the procedure, a bypass may have to be performed straight away during the person's stay in hospital).

So for some people (like Robin below), stents can solve the problem very effectively, but for others, like Margaret, the atherosclerosis is so pronounced that, even with a stent in place, the artery will become blocked again. This happens in approximately 10–30 per cent of cases, and for these people it may mean another angioplasty or, as in Margaret's case, a heart bypass operation.

Robin

One person who has had a hospital experience of angioplasty with stent is Robin. He is a council deputy chief executive in his early sixties. His life is stressful and, as he admits himself, he is a bit overweight and doesn't take enough exercise. He knows these factors can increase the risk of developing heart disease, but he points out in his defence that he doesn't smoke, and on most days he walks about half a mile to and from work. He first began to notice chest pains while walking on his way back from work, and these would only go away if he stopped for a moment and took a few deep breaths. After a couple of months he went to see his GP who suggested that this was almost certainly angina and that there was probably a problem with his coronary arteries.

Robin was prescribed a glyceryl trinitrate spray, which relieved the pain very effectively, and was then referred to a consultant cardiologist. He was given several preliminary tests, including blood tests which showed his total cholesterol to be higher than desirable at 5.7 mmol/L; and his blood pressure was also too high at around 170/90. He was given both a resting and stress ECG, an echocardiogram, and an angiogram (see Chapter 4 for descriptions of these tests). The angiogram identified two blocked coronary arteries and it was decided to carry out an angioplasty during which stents would be inserted into the blocked arteries.

'I was carted down to a cardiac area, a cardiac catheter unit for angiograms, angioplasties and stent procedures, with people lying around either having had this sort of treatment or waiting for it ... None of them seemed in dire circumstances and the staff were reassuring in that it all seemed so matter-of-fact ... They give you a little local anaesthetic before they put the catheter in – they used the same site as they had used for the angiogram and they plugged it with a collagen plug after the catheter was withdrawn ... you have to carry a card with you for three months in case you have an accident and someone else is thinking of using the same site ... They also put me on something called clopidogrel [an anti-platelet drug]. I stayed on the aspirin – I stay on that for ever! I was on clopidogrel before the procedure and for six months afterwards. What they said was that the big complication of this procedure is clotting, so they've got two things to prevent that. One is the clopidogrel, with the aspirin too, of course, and the other thing is that they used something called drug-eluting stents.

'I felt absolutely nothing during the procedure. The main discomfort was when removing the catheter after the stenting procedure but nothing really. The whole thing only took around half an hour. When they got to the blocked part they inflated the balloon . . . the thing that impresses me in retrospect is how they were finding their way around this great maze. It's all very calm and casual but there must be tremendous skill involved. In the end the doctor put in four stents – I think three in one artery and one in another – and when this had all been done, you could see the dye flowing through freely. Where there had been this gap in the flow it was now all connected up. What he then showed me, which was nice, after it was all finished, was a 'before and after' image on the monitor, just like a big 'home TV screen'. He showed how the coronary arteries were before the procedure and how they were afterwards.'

Robin stayed overnight in the hospital and went home the next day. He was put on 25 mg atenolol (a beta blocker), 40 mg simvastatin to help control his cholesterol, and 75 mg aspirin once a day to prevent clotting. He was also given advice about exercise and diet. His total cholesterol came down to 3.6 mmol/L and his blood pressure, which he now monitors himself, is generally around or under 120/75.

He added: 'I felt fine afterwards . . . We went down to the seaside about a month after it was done and I said to my wife, "Let's go up the cliff a bit." She said, "You can't do that!" And it's perfectly true, I wouldn't have been able to before. But I walked up there with no trouble at all!'

Heart bypass (coronary bypass surgery)

Heart bypass operations are performed in order to find a way around (i.e. to bypass) a narrowed part of a coronary artery, as can be seen in Figure 4, reproduced from the excellent booklet *Coronary Angioplasty and Coronary Bypass Surgery* from the Heart Information Series produced by the British Heart Foundation.

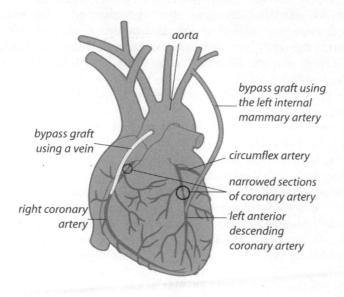

aorta

bypass graft using
the left internal
mammary artery

bypass graft
using a vein

circumflex artery

narrowed sections
of coronary artery

right coronary
artery

left anterior
descending
coronary artery

Figure 4 Coronary bypass surgery

In order to find a way around the narrowed coronary artery the surgeon has to take a blood vessel from somewhere else in the body and then graft this at one end to the aorta, which is the main artery leaving the heart, and at the other end to a part of the coronary artery beyond the blockage. In Figure 4 it can be seen that one of the grafts involves the use of a vein (this is usually the saphenous vein taken from the leg, although occasionally the radial artery in the arm is used) and the other graft has used the internal mammary artery from the chest. Typically, those having bypass surgery will need between one and five arteries bypassed. You may even find light-hearted competition between those having bypasses about the number they had to have: from 'just a triple bypass' to 'they were so bunged up, they had to do a quadruple bypass' and then to a 'top patient' like Peter (Chapter 1) who needed five coronary bypasses!

The type of bypass approach just described is called Coronary Artery Bypass Grafting or CABG (often referred to as 'Cabbage'!). It is carried out under general anaesthetic. To get at the heart, the first thing the surgeon has to do is to make a vertical incision down the breast bone (the sternum) and divide it to expose the heart. At the same time, the blood vessel to be used in the graft will be removed in readiness for the graft. One advantage of using an internal mammary artery is that these blood vessels tend to last longer without becoming obstructed and narrowed.

During the op the person will be placed on a heart-lung machine which takes over the functions of the heart artificially and ensures that a good supply of oxygenated blood continues to circulate around the body. While this machine is doing the heart's work, the surgeon can stop the heart for a short time in order to carry out the grafts more easily. When the grafts have been completed, the heart will be restarted, and as soon as it begins to function normally, the person will be taken off the heart-lung machine, the sternum is knitted together with wire sutures, and the chest and leg wounds are closed with sutures or clips. Then the person is taken to intensive care, and usually stays there for a couple of days. In most cases, people leave the hospital within a week or so, although it will usually take around three months to get over the operation properly. We discuss various approaches to post-bypass rehabilitation in Chapters 9 to 14.

Risks and coronary bypass surgery

All surgery carries *some* risk, of course, and bypass surgery is no exception. The risk of serious complications depends upon several factors, including the state of your health before surgery. Remember, however, that for people in need of bypass surgery, the risks of dying or suffering further complications such as an MI or a stroke during the surgical procedure itself are extremely small compared with the risks of continuing *without bypass surgery*. You can check the mortality rates for bypass operations carried out in different hospitals (they're usually between 0 per cent and 2 per cent), but it's important to bear in mind that the mortality rates in *specialist* hospitals dealing with the most serious cases will be inflated to some extent because of the more complicated health problems of those with whom they are dealing.

Less invasive bypass procedures

In some cases, less 'invasive' bypass procedures are able to be used. One technique is called Minimally Invasive Direct Coronary Artery Bypass (or MIDCAB) and this can be performed without a heart-lung bypass machine and without opening the breast bone (hence the use of the term 'minimally invasive').

What happens is that a small incision is made above the diseased coronary artery and one of the mammary arteries supplying the chest will normally be used to effect a bypass. Only one to two bypasses can be carried out during such an operation, although balloon angioplasty can be performed at the same time. The main advantage of this type of operation is that it does not require the use of a heart-lung machine.

Another procedure is called beating-heart surgery, also sometimes referred to as off-pump coronary bypass surgery or OPCAB. This involves using special techniques that keep part of the heart still, so that the surgeon can operate on two or more coronary arteries without having to stop the heart completely. The breast bone still has to be opened to gain access in this method, but the heart-lung bypass machine is not required – though it is always kept on standby.

One advantage of the less invasive procedures is that they help to minimize the degree of 'collateral' damage to tiny blood vessels in the brain that can sometimes occur during a bypass operation. This damage is caused by minute pieces of 'debris', such as bits of plaque which become detached from the artery walls. These bits of debris can then flow through the blood vessels from the heart and into the brain. The debris usually becomes detached from the artery walls as a result of the use of surgical clamps. In any major operation, surgical clamps are used to block off blood vessels while the surgeons are working on the body's internal organs.

During bypass surgery various arteries are clamped in order to allow the doctors to perform the 'recoupling' operation in which the new vessels are grafted on to healthy arteries to bypass those that are diseased. (This process, by which the blood supply is restored to the coronary arteries, is sometimes referred to as coronary artery revascularization.) Unfortunately, if a clamp is used on a section of an artery that is badly diseased and in which the atherosclerotic plaque is very hard and brittle, this can result in little bits of detached plaque finding their way into the tiny blood vessels of the brain. If this debris blocks any of these tiny blood vessels this can produce a very small blockage in which part of the brain is starved of blood.

The areas of the brain most frequently affected are those concerned with memory and thinking (often called 'cognitive functioning') and, in general, temporary memory loss is the most common symptom. In Stephen's case, for example, it's possible that some of the temporary memory lapses he experienced might have been related to this phenomenon – but his memory was back to normal in a few weeks (see page 34). Occasionally areas of the brain relating to personality characteristics such as placidity or irritability may also be involved.

Fortunately, techniques are now available that allow surgeons to control the extent of this collateral damage by reducing the amount of the debris reaching the brain. In particular, they are able to distinguish between those parts of a diseased artery that are relatively safe to clamp and those that are less safe, when examined from the viewpoint of their propensity for producing particles of shattered plaque. It is also possible for the surgical team to monitor the brain to check whether such particles have reached it.

This is done by using a Doppler machine, a type of ultrasound scanner, which can identify HITS (High Intensity Transient Signals) which indicate that plaque particles have reached the brain. So different bypass techniques can now be assessed by reference to the number of HITS they produce. However, unlike the pop music industry, the fewer the number of HITS the surgeons manage to produce the better!

In David's case (described in Chapter 1), in addition to his quadruple bypass, the surgeon also performed something called an endarterectomy, in which an incision is made above the narrowed part of an artery and the plaque 'scraped out'. This is often carried out on the carotid artery which feeds blood to the brain, and then it is called carotid endarterectomy. There are two other treatments for clearing obstructions in the coronary arteries but these are not yet widely available in the UK. These are laser angioplasty, which follows the usual angioplasty approach, but uses a laser instead of a balloon at the tip of the catheter; and rotational atherectomy, in which a very small revolving drill is placed at the end of a catheter and effectively drills out the plaque.

The hospital experiences of bypass surgery as described by David and Peter

These comments are based on interviews with David and Peter, whose cases are described in Chapter 1.

David again
David went in for his bypass following many years in which he had suffered from painful angina. After his angiogram, the consultant came round to see him and said: 'Most of your coronary arteries are blocked. Your heart muscle is working

pretty well but you need to have a quadruple bypass operation as soon as possible. You're a very fit man apart from your blocked arteries, but if you don't have the operation I couldn't give you more than six months.' While he waited for a call from the teaching hospital, David carried on with his usual gardening activities, mowing the lawn and going on regular walks despite his angina, but his GP kept a check on him and supervised his medication closely until, after several months, he was eventually admitted for the operation.

On admission to hospital, as David puts it: 'No time was wasted by the efficient staff who put me through a whole battery of tests. After I was given the pre-med I remembered nothing. The next thing I can remember, but only hazily, is catheters and tubes being removed from various parts of my anatomy and a distant voice saying – "This will feel a bit funny for a moment or two but don't worry" – and then I drifted off to sleep again. After I woke up next morning (as I imagined) I was given tea and some breakfast and encouraged to get up and "try a little walk". This I performed energetically for some time, causing the charge nurse to remark that I was quite the "star patient". I replied that I felt very well, but wondered whether I shouldn't be getting ready for my op. "I shouldn't worry about that, David, you had it two days ago!" he said. I had some problems with my heart rate becoming fast and irregular (they called it "atrial fibrillation") but the doctors and nurses dealt with it all very calmly and expertly.

'I couldn't face any food for nearly a week and had to make a real effort to drink even a little fluid. Consequently the body's normal elimination processes slowed right down . . . I lost weight and I had become rather dehydrated and weak as a kitten. But I was reasonably comfortable in a dozy, listless sort of way . . . I had a bit of a dry, sore throat – I think a result of the tubes put down my throat during the op – and this made my voice a bit strange, like a voice from a distant shore!

'Before discharge we were warned about the possibility of changes in mood, depression, "good and bad days", "looking for improvements over weeks rather than days" . . . A number of people did have bouts of depression while in hospital, but I seemed to cope without any emotional upheaval . . . A friend of mine who had one artery unblocked couldn't walk the width between two lamp posts before the op. Afterwards he could walk without difficulty. But he suffered depression for about a month after the op . . . He's been fine since, though.'

David was kept on his beta blocker (atenolol), a cholesterol-lowering drug (simvastatin) and low-dose aspirin, prescribed painkillers to take as and when necessary, and was discharged from hospital after about ten days.

'We were given walking exercise in the hospital and very comprehensive printed instructions on exercise and lifestyle for when we got home – "no driving for at least six weeks, try to walk an additional 100 metres each day, but not if cold or wet, don't lift anything weighing over 10 lbs for the first three months" ... They told me I must start walking – and I did. I enjoyed it. My leg (the one they'd taken the vein from) was a bit painful. Heart no trouble at all – but the leg pain was a bit cramp-like ... The doctor suggested I could walk round and round the garden but I thought that was a bit boring. So I walked round the lanes in the village. I set myself goals, like getting to a certain tree, or lamp post one day and reaching one further up the road the next.'

Peter again

Peter, the other person described in Chapter 1, had five coronary bypasses during his operation. He was surprised at how coronary heart disease had crept up on him: 'I'd never had any problems. No chest pains, no faintness. But the arteries were all furred up. It's worrying to think how long the build-up had been going on and I'd been quite unaware of it!'

When he was in hospital he just left it all to the staff. He was impressed by the treatment he received and the way they controlled pain: 'There was no pain after the op. They encouraged me to get out of bed as soon as I was back in the ward from intensive care ... Later on the physiotherapists came round. They wanted me to try walking up some steps. They seemed pleased with my progress and said I could go home in a couple of days' time.'

During his stay of six days in hospital, the only problems he encountered were minor: 'The adhesive plaster was a bit itchy, and my leg ached a bit, but the stitches and clips they put in didn't hurt at all. If I was talking to someone who was going to have a bypass operation and was a bit worried about it, I'd say, "Go for it" – it's the best thing you can do ... Just leave it to the experts. They know what they're doing and you're in good hands.'

He was put on sotalol (a beta blocker) to lower his blood pressure and control arrhythmias, low-dose aspirin to thin the blood, and simvastatin to keep his cholesterol in check. 'I was also given a nitrate spray, but I've never had to use it because I've never really had any chest pains ... About six weeks after the op my leg swelled up – I'd developed a blood clot. But they sorted me out at the hospital and I've never had any further problems, except the odd ache in the leg every now and then ... I've also had a few arrhythmias when my heart has started to beat very fast ... "tachycardia". But I've gone straight to the hospital each time and they've sorted it out for me. A bit like taking your car into the garage when it's ticking over too fast. The mechanics know what they're up to and get it back into rhythm in no time!'

Peter also knew that if these arrhythmias became a bit of a nuisance, the doctors could easily sort this out with a pacemaker – a tiny piece of equipment that is implanted under the skin, usually in the upper left side of the chest, and helps to keep the heart rate regular. He was entirely happy to leave his treatment to the hospital doctors who had dealt so successfully with his heart bypass.

9

Going home

Following surgery, you will be looking forward to going back to your own home comforts, your own bed and your privacy! When recovering from routine cardiac surgery you will normally be physically independent, and able to walk, climb stairs, dress yourself and perform light domestic tasks. Most people will feel reasonably positive at this stage, perhaps even elated. There is a feeling of relief that the surgery is over and anticipation at the news that you are ready to come home.

But there is also likely to be some anxiety, including concern about being out of hospital so soon after surgery. You have the reassurance, though, of knowing that back-up local services are on hand to help you regain your fitness and to achieve a good post-bypass quality of life. With such help, most people are amazed at how quickly they start feeling better.

Different phases of rehabilitation

There are many ways of classifying the different phases of rehabilitation (or recovery) after a bypass operation. But we have chosen three broad phases which encompass most of the points you will need to think about after your discharge from hospital. These are:

- Recuperating at home during the first six weeks or so after discharge.
- Taking part in a cardiac rehabilitation programme usually lasting between eight and twelve weeks.
- Developing longer-term self-management strategies.

We will deal with the second and third phases in later chapters, but we start in this chapter with your post-operative recovery at home.

Going home from hospital

The first thing that has to be organized is your journey home, and you will need to have a travelling companion. If you are travelling by car you will find it useful to protect your chest from the seat belt by using a small folded towel as a 'cushion'. You may find that you want to break up a long road journey by taking a few stops to allow you to walk around a bit. If you're travelling by train, you need to try to ensure that you don't have to cope with too many steps, and you should also make sure that it's your companion who is carrying the bags!

When you're ready to leave the hospital, the staff will normally give you two copies of a 'discharge' letter: one for you to keep, and the other to give to your GP. This will give details about the operation you have had and mention any special requirements (e.g. blood tests, removal of stitches) and it will list your medication. Any dressings you are likely to require will usually have been organized with the district nurse before you leave.

You may also be given a discharge leaflet giving advice on how to look after yourself when you get home, covering the sorts of concerns we discuss later in this chapter. You are likely to receive details of heart support groups available in your area and to be advised that someone from your local cardiac rehabilitation team will be in touch – and from this point on, it will be your GP and local rehabilitation services that will take primary responsibility for your care.

One local cardiac rehabilitation nurse co-ordinator describes what happens in her area: 'The referral is usually faxed to us on the day of discharge. We ring the person as soon as that fax arrives – to make contact so they know who we are, to give them our telephone number, to identify if there are any immediate problems, and we ask standard questions – e.g. are your wounds OK, are you having any district nurse input, are your ankles swollen, are you eating, are you sleeping, is your pain controlled? Anything that's an issue at that early stage is usually very simple to remedy, e.g. by getting a district nurse to treat a wound that has become infected or started to weep.

'We always go and see a patient within a week of discharge. They nearly always need a couple of days to get over the journey home and just to find their feet and settle down. If you meet them at the door as soon as they get back from hospital they haven't had a chance to get into their routine and see what's a problem and what's not. We work as a multi-disciplinary team and when you work in a specific area you get to know your district and practice nurses very well because you're liaising with them all the time.'

Despite all the excellent support staff available, however, the person best able to get you motivated to begin your rehabilitation programme in an enthusiastic and positive manner is *you*! Much will depend on your self-belief in your ability to improve your fitness, to make lifestyle changes and to adjust emotionally following surgery.

This view is well articulated by Margaret (whose case is described in Chapter 4): 'The recovery time is up to you really, because the more you want to get better, the more you follow the rehab programme and that helps you recover.'

Adjusting to being at home again and setting goals

This initial period of adjusting to being home and settling into a routine is important as this initiates good 'habits' and structure. Being bored, having little structure in your day or week, fewer social outings and less physical activity than you are used to, will soon start to make your rehabilitation seem uncertain and uninteresting. But by giving yourself small goals in the early stages, based on the advice you have received on discharge, you can begin to build up your confidence and sense of achievement. David (page 60) illustrates this point very well. You may remember how he gradually built up the length of his daily walk around the village. He set himself goals, such as reaching a particular tree or lamp post on one day, and then challenged himself to reach a more distant one on the next day.

Robert (see Chapter 10) explains how he set himself special targets, one of which was to walk to the hairdresser's and back: 'It's not all that far, but I always used to drive before I had the op. It's a good target to set, because it's attainable on my walking schedule.' He might also have added that it will soon become a necessity unless he changes his hairstyle from short, to long back and sides!

He also describes his aim to walk to other parts of the town he'd never visited before. He followed the hospital's instructions assiduously, adding a minute each day to his five-minute 'starter' walk: 'I started doing things I wouldn't have dreamt of doing when I was working – like window shopping, and having a cup of coffee in town. I never had time to do this sort of thing before. I was always rushing around, chasing my tail. I rather enjoyed these new experiences. They acted as rewards for all the effort I was putting in building up my exercise levels . . . It's an odd experience, though. I always used to be in the fast lane, a brisk walker, never slow. Now I was being overtaken by elderly people with walking sticks! That was a bit depressing. But I could feel myself slowly beginning to accelerate. There's no way you can push it too much, though. Your body dictates the speed.'

Points of concern during the early weeks of recuperation

In the first few weeks you may be a bit apprehensive about how you will cope. But you will get an early visit from the cardiac nurse, as one nurse explains: 'People get one home visit from us. If they need more, then we will provide more, but on the whole most people are fine with one visit. They have our phone number and they can contact us and we very much encourage them to be taking charge and control of themselves. When we see them, if they're well and have no complications, we'll book them in for rehab close to six weeks after surgery. If we've not heard from them in two or three weeks, we assume all is well.'

You can expect one or two minor inconveniences during the early weeks, and will probably be a little anxious about what is normal and what is unusual. We list below a few pointers that might help you – but give your GP, practice or cardiac nurse a ring if you need extra advice.

Itching or numbness in your scars

As you will have noticed with small grazes to your skin, when parts of your body are healing they tend to itch, or sometimes to feel numb – and this is all part of the natural process of healing. The main advice is to avoid scratching! However, if a wound becomes swollen or painful or produces a discharge, you should contact your district nurse or GP. It's usually safe to wash the wounds daily, but do this gently with mild soap and warm water. You can take showers as soon as any stitching staples have been removed, but it's probably sensible to check with your district nurse first to make sure this is OK.

If the bypass involved taking a graft from your leg, follow the advice given to you by the nurses before you left hospital. This will usually involve advice to avoid standing or sitting for long periods in one position and not to cross your legs since this impairs circulation. The nurses are also likely to have advised you to raise your leg while sitting, e.g. resting the leg on a cushioned stool, to help circulation, and to contact the GP if your leg starts to swell up more than usual. If you were prescribed elastic stockings (like Peter, see page 69), you will have been advised to wear these during the day, for a couple of weeks or so, and to remove them at bedtime.

Pain control and other medication

You will be given a supply of 'painkillers' (analgesics) before you leave hospital, and you may need these for a little while after you get home. One of the problems with some analgesic tablets, however, is that they can make you constipated, so you may need to ensure that you have some good laxative foods to accompany them! Stephen (see Chapter 5) had this problem: 'Stopping the painkillers was a difficult decision because I wanted to be pain-free and I also wanted to go to the toilet! But the toilet won in the end. We had a bit of a laugh about it.' His wife, Helen, says: 'I was giving him all these prunes and figs and laxatives like Senokot. His tummy was just getting bigger and bigger, and he still couldn't go – and, of course, he wasn't supposed to strain on the loo! So in the end he just gave up the painkillers and went on to things like codeine, and eventually his bowels got back to normal.'

Some people express surprise that they are still on medication *after* their bypass. As Robert says: 'I'm a bit disconcerted that I'm still on tablets. I thought I might not need so many as before, but I'm still on the same number.' Each individual case is different, of course, and some people, like Sheila (page 108), *are* on fewer tablets after their bypass. The fact is, though, that even with the blood flowing nicely through the cardiovascular system, it's still necessary to 'fine tune' each individual's body so that the heart works as efficiently as possible and without too much effort. The GP explained to Robert that the tablets 'would keep his blood pressure down and were excellent as preventative treatment for angina'. Robert saw the sense in that: 'If it keeps me in good nick now and helps to stop me getting heart problems later on, I'll take the pills quite happily.'

Disturbed sleep and lack of appetite

When you get back home you'll almost certainly feel very tired but, at the same time, your normal sleeping pattern may be disturbed. You may also find you don't have much appetite to begin with – although the sight and smell of some familiar home cooking can soon remedy this! Such temporary disturbances are to be expected. Sometimes sleep disruption can be a consequence of taking daytime naps. Because you are feeling extra tired you may decide to have an afternoon 'cat nap', for example, and this can be quite 'restorative' – but if you sleep too long, it can disturb the pattern of your night-time sleep. It's a matter of finding the right balance. Some people also find that they experience one or two strange dreams after they get back home (usually only for a short time) and these probably result from the anaesthetic and medication used during the operation. For the same reason, you may experience some blurred vision at times, but again, this should settle down within a few weeks, as should any appetite problems.

Getting comfortable

One of the things you will find a bit difficult on first coming home is sorting out comfortable sleeping and sitting positions because of discomfort from various wounds. You'll need to experiment, but here are one or two people's tips. Robert says: 'If I was to recommend one thing, it would be to get a hot water bottle, or a heat pad'; and Stephen found it more comfortable sitting up in the bed with several pillows, rather than lying down:

'In hospital there was a thick rope attached to the end of the bed. You could just pull yourself up on it. It was brilliant. Because that's one of the most painful things to do without some assistance, raising yourself up to get out of bed. We don't have anything to attach a rope to, so I had to make do with tucking in the top sheet tightly at the bottom of the bed and pulling myself up with the sheet . . . It's also important that the chair you sit in isn't too low. Hauling yourself up out of a low chair can cause a lot of discomfort. You can get blocks or casters which raise the legs of chairs to a comfortable height.'

Finally, remember that loose-fitting clothes will be more comfortable than tight-fitting ones because they put much less strain on the sites of incisions.

Exercise and rest

Getting a good balance between exercise and rest is important in the first few weeks. The heart is a muscle, and we need to exercise it in order to keep it in good shape, but it's important to follow the guidelines you will be given about how much exercise to do; and it's equally important to include periods of rest so that your body is not overworked. You or your partner may need to dissuade friends and family from too many (or too lengthy) 'welcome home' visits. While it is nice to have this social contact, it's more important at the early stage of your recuperation that you are able to rest when you need to do so.

We discuss some specific exercises in Chapter 11, but you will probably be given a pamphlet on discharge which will get you started. Just remember the basic rule: do *not* exercise immediately after a meal when your body needs to concentrate on digesting the food you have eaten.

Because his lungs were still a bit congested (a common, short-term after-effect of the anaesthetic), Stephen also had another exercise – he had to practise coughing: 'The staff would roll up a towel and tape it, or hold it to your chest. You hold it against your chest and then force yourself to cough, starting with little coughs and building up. In this way it's manageable. You control the discomfort of coughing. But if you sneezed involuntarily without taking this sort of preparatory action, you'd go through the ceiling! I used the same towel method at home. It works really well.'

Lifting, pushing and pulling

It is particularly important to avoid any heavy lifting, pushing or pulling for at least six weeks. Basically, you should try to avoid any activity that will put a strain on the upper arms or chest. This means that you need to be careful, for example, about carrying shopping bags, using a vacuum cleaner, or reaching up and pulling down the boot of a car. You can lift a half-full kettle to make a cup of tea or coffee, but don't try lifting heavy saucepans straightaway.

Resuming sex

During sex our bodies are aroused and active, and it is estimated that during sexual intercourse with our usual partner in familiar surroundings, there is a rise in blood pressure and heart rate that is broadly equivalent to the levels we would experience if walking up two flights of stairs – and this sort of aerobic exercise is generally beneficial to heart-health (see Chapter 11). So you need to treat sex in the same way that you would treat any other activity that results in an increase in cardiovascular activity. Take it easy and pace yourself. It's also important that you adopt a comfortable position, and that you only resume your sex life when both you and your partner feel ready for it. This may be anywhere between three and four weeks to six weeks or longer.

Getting back to driving

The guidance issued by the DVLA indicates that you should not start to drive again for four weeks post-surgery, but people are generally advised to leave it for about six weeks. Your car insurance company should be informed that you have had a bypass, and for people with HGV or PSV licences it's necessary to inform the DVLA. One tip is offered by Stephen: 'I found it very helpful to put a thin cushion against my chest before putting the seat belt on in the car. It made it much more comfortable.'

Emotional reactions

Your mood may still be fluctuating from day to day. You may feel rather down and a bit irritable one day, emotional and tending to cry for no apparent reason another, but then quite happy or even elated at other times. These emotional 'ups and downs' are quite common for the first few weeks. Margaret tells how she felt on getting back from hospital: 'I had a little bit of depression for the first two months, especially the first month. For some reason, I just cried and I've no idea why. I was just feeling low. They warned me that it could happen . . . I said to myself, "That's it, finish it because if you keep on thinking about it the more you'll become depressed – and I don't want to be depressed" . . . Another time I could not read . . . as much as I wanted to, my concentration wasn't there . . . I didn't even feel like watching television – but I'm not one for sitting down a lot . . . I kept myself busy, doing the exercises they gave me, at home.'

But if the ups and downs go on longer than a few weeks, and you are worried about your emotional health, have a chat with your GP or cardiac nurse who will be able to offer advice. Sometimes people become low in mood because they are frustrated that they are not feeling fitter more quickly. If so, take time to reflect and remind yourself that you are on a journey to recovery, and that this journey is only just beginning. You need time to adapt, and you need to give yourself the space to adjust slowly and practically to the physical and emotional demands of your recovering body.

Getting used to friends and family helping out

For someone who has always been very independent and used to helping other people, it can be very difficult to make the adjustment to becoming to some extent dependent on others and being the recipient rather than the giver of help. Sheila (Chapter 14) describes her feelings: 'It's amazing how tired you are when you first come home, but the hardest thing I think is having to have someone to help you. I just couldn't get in and out of the bath, so my eldest granddaughter used to help me. Very brave she was 'cos she doesn't like scars and things.'

On the other hand, some people rather take to being 'mollycoddled' for a bit. Peter took this attitude both in hospital and at home. He suggests that people should 'sit back and relax and leave it to the experts . . . They know what they're doing.' In hospital the experts were the surgeons and nurses, but at home, as he readily acknowledges, the 'expert' was his wife who acted as his best friend, carer and nurse – and the biggest problem they had was 'getting the elasticated stockings on and off'!

Once you have arrived back home it's important that you try to be practical, keep a positive outlook and take the opportunities that will be available to you from your local cardiac rehabilitation service. We look at these in the next chapter.

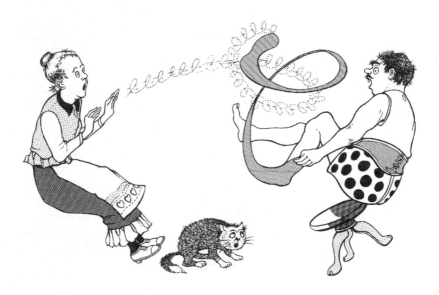

The biggest problem . . .

10
Cardiac rehabilitation programmes

Cardiac rehabilitation programmes usually offer group sessions supervised by health professionals and structured to aid your recovery. The rehab programmes are sometimes hospital-based and sometimes community-based (e.g. in a local leisure centre). You will have been given details about available programmes prior to your discharge. If it is appropriate for you to attend (and it usually is), the cardiac rehab co-ordinator will arrange for you to join one of the groups.

Although programmes differ from region to region, most programmes run for between eight and twelve weeks. The sessions usually start after about six weeks or so post-surgery, partly because this is when those who are post-bypass usually start driving again, which makes it easier to attend the sessions without having to rely on public transport or on the goodwill of family and friends. The sessions will provide you with an exercise class or programme that will be appropriate for your medical history and physical capabilities. There may also be some educational or lifestyle input (often a rolling programme that runs alongside the physical rehab classes) featuring seminars/talks from healthcare professionals such as dietitians, nursing staff, pharmacists and counsellors/psychologists. Topics can range from stress management and understanding your medicines, to surgical wound management.

Attendance at a rehab programme is not mandatory, but it is generally seen as one of the most beneficial aspects of your post-bypass care. Here are some of the comments made by a number of people who have seen the benefits of rehab programmes:

- 'They work you hard, but I enjoyed it. I thought it was very helpful.'
- 'I did eight weeks of rehab. I found all the gentlemen in the class very interesting because I was the only lady!'
- 'What's nice about the classes is you meet other people. I enjoyed it. It was lovely. I was really sorry to leave.'
- 'We used to meet before we went into class to have a coffee and if someone didn't turn up we worried about them. I just think we bonded because you're all in the same boat.'
- 'I did like the rehab because it made me feel good!'

It's natural for the main emphasis in rehab classes to be on your physical recovery, but emotional aspects are also covered. The co-ordinator of one well-organized rehab programme describes how they try to cover psychological elements: 'We have our own fully qualified counsellors who will offer home or clinic visits. [In other rehab settings this input may be provided by nurses/advisers or health psychologists.] They do three or four sessions in the rehab programme, including general relaxation, stress management and coping skills. They will also see people on their own, and with their partners.'

Although attendance at cardiac rehab sessions is voluntary, we would strongly advise you to take up the offer if at all possible. There is persuasive research evidence to show that people at the post-bypass stage can gain real physical and psychological benefit from cardiac rehabilitation programmes; and attendance at such courses is strongly advocated by the Department of Health and by leading heart associations such as the British Heart Foundation and the British Association of Cardiac Rehabilitation.

From talking to hospital staff and cardiac nurses, or from reading leaflets and books, you may feel you already have quite a good grasp as to what is required in order to make a good recovery from your operation – but attending a rehab programme will provide that extra dimension. There is no substitute for real interactions on a face-to-face basis with trained professionals involved with your care; and it is helpful to know that if problems or issues crop up unexpectedly, you will have a regular and easily accessible forum in which to discuss them.

If it is difficult for you to attend the sessions for any reason, the co-ordinators will usually be able to find ways of accommodating your requirements. The co-ordinator of one rehab programme comments that: 'We do have people that don't fit into normal cardiac rehab, e.g. they're elderly and infirm, they don't drive and so on. We can offer a seated exercise programme for them to do at home, and we try to be very flexible. For some of our elderly frail ladies, their only aim is to be able to walk to the shop and back. We've sent out our physio assistants in those first six weeks after they've come home, to go out with them, to get their confidence up to walk to the shops and back ... That becomes their rehab ...

'Some people just don't like the idea of the group session, so we've been developing home rehab programmes. Most of the circuits can be done at home – you can go up and down the bottom step of the stairs, you can hold two cans of something to do your bicep exercises, and so on; the exercise physiologists or physios teach people to take their pulses, to recognize their heart rate, and they follow them up on a weekly or two-weekly basis to see how they're progressing.'

So, even if you're experiencing problems in getting to the rehab sessions, don't despair, and don't write rehab off without first having a chat with the rehab co-ordinator. He or she will usually manage to find some way of providing you with appropriate support. Taking part in an individually tailored rehab programme will form a key part of your recovery and, despite a few initial reservations, people usually find that they actually like the opportunity of talking to other people who have had similar experiences: 'I found this very useful. You could ask people all sorts of questions you wouldn't bother your doctor with – "Have you had any trouble with your stitches? How's your leg? Does it still hurt a bit? Have you been on these tablets? Did you find they made you constipated?" . . . You find out that other people have had exactly the same problems that you've had, and you can discuss all sorts of things with them without embarrassment, knowing that they've been through the same experiences as you.'

We describe in the next chapter some of the main features of the sort of exercise programmes you will be advised to follow in the rehab sessions, together with advice on general lifestyle issues.

Robert

Robert is a self-employed graphic designer aged 58. He no longer has to support his grown-up family, but since his wife does not work, the two of them live solely on his income. They enjoy quite a reasonable standard of living, and are used to taking two or three holidays a year, at least one of them with their local rambling club. Robert jogs and cycles regularly and has always thought of himself as an extremely fit person. However, there is a family history of heart disease. His father had a sudden, fatal heart attack at the age of 78, and a post-mortem revealed that he had suffered from several previous small, apparently symptomless myocardial infarctions (so-called 'silent' MIs). Shortly after his father's death, Robert's mother also found out that what she believed to be 'acid indigestion' was actually pain from stable angina. She was put on a beta blocker for this and remained reasonably fit and active well into her eighties.

The shock of finding out about his father's cardiac problems prompted Robert to avail himself of a 'well person' check-up at his GP's surgery. He had put his father's problems down to heavy smoking and lack of exercise and he was not, therefore, expecting to find any problems with his own heart-health, since he was a non-smoker and keen on exercise. However, the check-up revealed that he *did* have problems with high blood pressure and raised cholesterol, but the results of a resting ECG test appeared normal. The doctor put him on 50 mg atenolol to lower his blood pressure, 40 mg provastatin to bring down his cholesterol, and 75 mg aspirin to thin his blood and help to prevent blood clots. He also advised him to try to keep to a cholesterol-lowering diet.

After this salutary health warning, Robert went for regular checks with his GP, and managed to get his blood pressure down to around 140/80 mm Hg and his cholesterol under 5.2 mmol/L. His GP was reasonably satisfied with these readings, and for the next five or so years Robert thought things were fine. However, on one of his rambling holidays in the Peak District he began to suffer from some strange symptoms. 'We were walking up a steep path and I became very short of breath. Then I started to get a feeling of a sort of reflux in the throat, and saliva coming into the mouth, and I had a heavy feeling in the shoulders and a thumping headache for a short while. Then it went off and I was OK . . . It was a bit of a shock, and as soon as we got back home I went back to the GP.'

Robert was put on 30 mg of lansoprazole for gastric reflux to see whether this would sort things out. But whenever he did anything that was physically demanding, such as jogging, the symptoms kept returning and his GP decided to refer him to a consultant cardiologist to check whether his symptoms might be angina. A stress ECG showed distinct abnormalities which the cardiologist said were likely to be caused by narrowing of the coronary arteries. Robert was placed on a waiting list for an angiogram and prescribed a nitrate spray to help with the angina pain.

The angiogram revealed several blockages. According to the consultant, he had 'one completely blocked artery and the others between 20 and 90 per cent blocked, with the left side critical'. He was informed that he would need heart surgery, and was immediately put on the waiting list for a bypass.

He took a proactive approach to the wait and focused on his fitness, and also spent time trying to think 'about all eventualities and everybody and everything that's going to be affected – my partner, my business, our leisure pursuits, everything. I've got a real problem with the business because I'm self-employed and I haven't got a 'critical illness' insurance. I should have had one, I know, but you never think something like this is going to happen to you when you're still several years off retirement.' He was worried that if he wasn't able to keep to his usual work schedule he'd lose some of his regular customers. 'So that's added a lot of stress . . . The fact that they've got me into hospital quickly is good in one way, but it's difficult in another because it hasn't given me enough time to sort out the jobs in hand, or the books.'

Robert was in hospital for eight nights. 'I quite enjoyed the first day . . . everyone was so helpful and considerate. I felt like a bit of a star! The next morning I had a bath and I was given all the preliminary treatments – antiseptics, pre-meds, that sort of thing – and after that I don't really remember a thing until my wife came in to see me.' By this time, Robert was out of intensive care and in the high dependency unit, but he still had all the usual trappings – linked up to all sorts of machines. His wife was prepared for this, but still found it upsetting. As Robert says, 'She's been through the shredder over this business. Probably more worried about it than I was. And when she came to see me first of all, I wasn't in much of a position to give her the reassurance she needed. I'd just had a quadruple bypass and I was still out of it!'

She perked up as she saw Robert making good improvement on the ward and was surprised how quickly he was up and walking again. When he got home he felt very tired and found it difficult to concentrate. 'I felt very fragile, but it was nice to be home again. At first I just wanted to cuddle a hot-water bottle all the time! . . . Funnily enough, I didn't want physical contact from my wife early on. My body felt too shattered – my chest was tight, my skin was very sensitive. It was worst at night. I couldn't sleep very well, but the hot-water bottle was a godsend. Now, my wife has started to replace the hot-water bottle but it took a few weeks!'

Robert went to see his GP, who reviewed his medication. This was similar to the pre-bypass regime, except that it now included an additional daily dose of 50 mg losartan, for blood pressure control (see page 26). He also received a visit from the cardiac nurse, who reserved him a place on a rehabilitation programme at the local leisure centre. Robert describes his approach to the 'training circuit' in this way: 'I pushed myself too hard at first . . . But I've got it well sorted now. I just gradually increase the amount I do each time . . . There's a bit of support from the sidelines, because people bring their partners along . . . they act like cheer-leaders. We get seminars in the afternoon, after exercising in the morning, but we're so whacked out we tend to drop off! . . . We had a talk on resuscitation – that made some people get a bit apprehensive, thinking they were going to need it themselves. But I thought of it as a useful training – something that I could use in emergency with someone else. I didn't think I was going to be in need of it. In fact, that shows how much better I was feeling.'

He likes setting himself goals, and competing against himself rather than others: 'I tend to treat life like a sport. I prepare for things, and try to have strategies and to set positive but achievable targets – like I'm aiming to have a good holiday this summer.' By next year he said he was planning to get back to rambling, and eventually skiing again: 'I'm not striving competitively, just to be able to take part will be a terrific result.'

Since the op, Robert's immediate 'game plan' was to get driving as soon as possible: 'I'm itching to get driving again. It's one of the things I was most concerned about before the op – I even went out at three o'clock in the morning to have a final drive the night before I went in!'

In the event, Robert was back driving within five weeks. He also went on a month's holiday with his wife, and on his return started working again part-time. Although still on sickness benefit, he was allowed to work for 16 hours a week, and was chuffed to get back to his job so soon. Robert asked a colleague to help him out until he was able to get back to work full-time. This enabled him to complete the jobs in hand and to keep his regular customers happy. As for his cherished dream of getting back on to the ski slopes, he paced his preparation carefully and, to his great delight, was back skiing within a year of his bypass operation.

11
Exercise and other lifestyle changes

One big advantage of attending cardiac rehab, as we have mentioned, is that your exercise will be supervised by expert professional staff such as physiotherapists, exercise physiologists and cardiac nurses. There is also something of a bonus if these are held in a community setting rather than hospital. According to one physiotherapist: 'If you can get people coming to a sports centre, there's every chance they'll continue attending activity sessions later on.' The suggestions on exercise that we offer in this chapter are no substitute for individual programmes designed by the professionals, but they will help to give you an idea of approaches you can adopt. It's a good idea, though, to check first with your physio, or the cardiac or practice nurse, to make sure that they're OK for you.

The exercises you will be advised to do when you're just back home (and later on as part of your normal exercise routines) are stretching exercises designed to prevent stiffness in those areas of your body that are tight after your surgery. These exercises will also help to improve circulation and promote good healing.

Warming up and cooling down

It is important to build up your level of exercise slowly, and before each session to warm up for between five and ten minutes so that your body is not taken by surprise! Some good warm-up exercises can be carried out either standing in a good upright posture (or sitting up straight on a chair or on the edge of the bed). When you are in a comfortable position, tilt your head towards one shoulder until you feel your neck stretching, then hold for five to ten seconds, repeat a couple of times, and then do the same tilting towards the opposite shoulder. You can also do the same sort of exercise with a rotation movement to one side and then the other. You may have seen athletes doing this type of warm-up routine as they are preparing themselves for the start of a sprint.

If you are sitting on a chair, you can also raise each leg in turn so that it is roughly parallel to the floor, then try to raise your toes towards your body, and hold this position for five to ten seconds, before slowly relaxing your leg and bringing your foot down to the floor again. You can also do a similar exercise with your arms – again, standing or sitting on a chair, extend one arm at a time (hand facing down), and pull your fingers of the extended arm back towards your body with the other hand, hold for five to ten seconds and then relax. Also, if your chest isn't too uncomfortable, you can try turning your chest gently from side to side to keep the upper part of your body flexible.

When you have done your warm-up, you might then do your regular exercise (e.g. brisk walking or cycling), and after any brisk exercise do a five- to ten-minute 'cool-down' to allow your pulse and breathing rates to return to normal. The cool-down may consist, for example, of walking slowly at the end of your proper walk or doing a few gentle stretching exercises. A good approach if you're using 'brisk walking' as your main exercise is to start your walk at a steady pace, then gradually increase this to a good 'brisk' pace, and finally, as you get to the end of your walk, to reduce your pace to slow walking, so that your heart rate and breathing are back to normal by the time you return home.

One exercise physiologist suggests a cool-down of five minutes' gentle stroll around the room, followed by stretching, to get the heart rate down from exercising levels, rather than just stopping abruptly, which can present difficulties for the blood to get back up to the heart.

Exercises in the rehab gym

When you enrol for cardiac rehab you'll find that you will be checked out at some sort of Induction session. As one exercise physiologist explains: 'Details are taken of weight, blood pressure and medication, and the person is put through what's called a "walk shuttle test" based on a "bleep" test designed for sportsmen and sportswomen, but modified for cardiac patients ... There's a 10-metre line and people have to walk from one end to the other before the "bleep". They are wired up to check heart rate, and to begin with they have 20 seconds to get from end to end. Then the time limit is gradually reduced. Finally, we check the levels achieved and design an appropriate programme for each individual.'

The basic fitness and stamina exercises are *aerobic* exercises that improve fitness through increased oxygen consumption, as in brisk walking (rather than *isometric* exercises, which involve straining, as in weight-lifting). So most rehab programmes will include activities like brisk shuttle walking, cycling, step-ups, mini-trampolining on a 'rebounder' ('a bit like a bouncy walk', as one member of rehab staff described it), or repeated standing up from sitting down. These will then be interspersed with less strenuous exercises that allow the person to recover in between the main activities (similar in exertion to the warm-up exercises we have already discussed). *Remember, though, that these exercises are not competitions.* You may feel like trying to compete with other members of the group, but it's best to resist this urge. Your exercise programme is individual, and the only person you are meant to be competing against is yourself!

Level of exertion

Before your exercise you will probably be asked to take your 'resting heart rate' by taking your pulse. The number of beats in one minute gives your resting heart rate (a quick way is to count the beats in 15 seconds and then multiply by 4). When you have finished exercising, the rehab staff will expect your pulse to be within 10 beats per minute of the resting rate. The staff will also establish what your *maximal heart rate* is, and in general it is advised that your heart rate during exercise should not reach more than 60–75 per cent of the maximal rate.

The usual formula for calculating maximal heart rate is to subtract your age from 220 (the maximal heart rate for a 20-year-old). So if you are 60 years old, then your maximal heart rate will be 160 and your heart rate should not rise above 60–75 per cent of this rate (i.e. it should keep within 96 to 120 beats per minute). Sometimes this rate needs to be adjusted further, to take account of general level of fitness, or any medication you may be taking that can affect your heart rate. As one physiologist explains, 'For instance, beta blockers slow down the pulse so we set a target lower for someone on these drugs.'

Another way of assessing level of exertion is by a 'rating of perceived exertion' (RPE). There are various ways of measuring this and the rehab staff will advise about their own approach. But they will range from a *low* level of perceived exertion during which exercise feels easy and effortless with no increased breathing rate, to *medium* acceptable levels in which you first begin to breathe a bit harder and feel warm, and then become a bit out of puff, but you are still able to talk comfortably. You should aim to go beyond the *low* level of exertion, but avoid reaching the *higher* levels of exertion in which you become so breathless that you can't speak, and your chest starts to tighten up.

The rehab staff will help you to recognize what is an appropriate exercise regime for you. One physiologist sums up the professionals' role: 'The whole point of us being here is to empower people and help them get their independence back, and the most important feedback we get is their build-up in confidence. When they first come to us they're very unsure about how far they should be going with exercise, and once they've gone through the programme with us, then their confidence returns.'

Getting back to regular exercise

You'll need to build up your body's capacity for physical exercise gradually. It's important to pace yourself, but now that your heart is able to function so much better than it was before the bypass, you should ultimately be able to achieve good levels of fitness. One question often asked by sports enthusiasts is whether they will be able to get back to playing sport again. The answer is usually 'yes' provided it's not a particularly strenuous form of activity – but it's always best to ask your rehab staff about this. If, for example, you played golf before your bypass, then you should certainly be able to play afterwards. You'll need to allow your body to heal sufficiently so that you can perform the sort of stretching and trunk-turning movements involved in golf without discomfort. One physio advises those golfers who are post-bypass to 'try putting or chipping a few balls first . . . don't get your "Big Bertha" golf club out and start driving hard. Then try four holes only with your friends . . . build it up slowly.' Without the handicap of unhealthy coronary arteries, you may even find that your post-bypass 'golfing handicap' actually improves! When you are back to regular exercise, then you should follow the usual guidelines for maintaining a healthy heart – these are to exercise at a medium, 'breathing hard' level for about 30 minutes, five days a week.

Watching your weight – the Body Mass Index (BMI)

Keeping yourself in trim is largely a matter of eating healthily (see next chapter) as well as exercising regularly; if your output in terms of energy expended matches your calorific intake, then you are likely to remain in good shape. To help you check that your weight is OK, you can use something called the Body Mass Index, calculated by the formula: weight in kilograms ÷ height in metres squared. So, if you weigh 64 kilograms (10 stones) and you are 1.68 metres (5 foot 6 inches) tall, your BMI will be $64 \div 1.68^2 = 22.7$.

In general, a BMI rating of less than 20 means that you are 'underweight', 20–24.9 is acceptable, 25–29.9 is overweight, and 30–40 is obese. It's not a perfect measure, and doesn't distinguish, for example, between men and women or between active and less active people. But it will give you an idea of whether you are underweight or overweight. To make it easy for you, we have provided a BMI chart (Figure 5 on page 82). Simply check your weight against your height measurement, and then the point at which these intersect will indicate your BMI rating.

Other lifestyle measures

Two other measures that are particularly important are eating healthily and keeping control of your stress levels. We look specifically at these issues in Chapters 12 and 14 respectively, but in this chapter we concentrate on looking at one other lifestyle change that many people will face – the need to stop smoking.

This is often the most essential (and in many cases the most difficult) lifestyle change that people need to make in order to give themselves the best chance of making a full recovery from heart disease.

Help is available from your GP, the rehab staff or from associations like the British Heart Foundation, QUIT and ASH (see page 120). Detailed advice is also given in *How to Keep Your Cholesterol in Check* by Robert Povey (Sheldon Press), but here are a few general hints to help you quit the habit:

- First, convince yourself that you need to stop smoking. A good place to start is to think about the major role that smoking has almost certainly played in leading to your cardiac problems and the need for a heart bypass.
- A good preparation for starting to quit is to write down all the positive advantages of quitting smoking – your improved health and wealth will do as a good starter for your list.
- Try to find a companion who is also keen to stop smoking and will work with you on the road to becoming a non-smoker – this will help to keep you both on track and give you valuable support in the process.

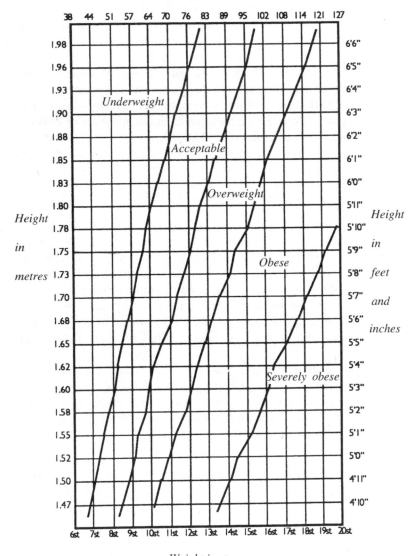

Figure 5 Body Mass Index (BMI) chart

- Although nicotine ensnares smokers with a powerful physical dependency, remember that the more you resist, the easier it becomes to resist.
- Try to avoid placing yourself in situations that tend to trigger your urge to smoke, and be willing to change your routines to avoid those trigger points.
- Replace your cigarette with something edible like a piece of fruit or a stick of carrot, or try chewing some sugar-free gum.
- Don't try to convince yourself that the odd cigarette won't matter – that 'odd cigarette' will put you back on the slippery slope!
- Compare notes regularly with your companion, and reward yourselves for your success.

Finally, as a mnemonic to help you remember the main points in adopting healthy lifestyle changes, we encourage you to **BE POSITIVE**!

Be sure to take your prescribed medication.
Exercise sensibly, following your rehab guidelines.

Pace yourself and remember that cardiac rehabilitation isn't a race!
Only drink alcohol in moderation (see guidelines in Chapter 12).
Smoking and smoky places should be avoided; instead, fill your lungs with fresh air.
Include time for hobbies and relaxation.
Take care to keep stress levels down (Chapter 14).
Involve your family and friends in making lifestyle changes with you.
Variations in weight should be kept within the recommended BMI (see page 82).
Eat healthily – keep low in fat, sugar, salt, and in the Glycaemic Index (see Chapter 12).

12
Eating for a healthy heart

As we have noted in Chapter 3, poor diet is one of the key risk factors for heart disease. Eating a healthy diet not only plays a significant role in preventing heart disease (see British Heart Foundation booklet, *Eating for Your Heart*), but it can also help to improve your heart's functioning after you have had your bypass. So in addition to feeling healthier, you will also be helping to prevent the need for further treatment. The approach we recommend is not a 'denial' regime in which you are asked to give up certain types of food; rather, it urges you to eat a whole range of tasty and enjoyable foods that are good for your heart, (Another Sheldon Press book, *Eating for a Healthy Heart*, by Povey, Morrell and Povey, explains the principles of healthy eating in more detail and includes over 90 delicious heart-healthy recipes.) To help you to establish a heart-healthy approach to eating and drinking, we summarize below some of the main guidelines:

- *Aim to eat at least five portions of fruit and vegetables per day*

Diets rich in fruit and vegetables have been found to lower the risk of heart disease. It is thought that this is partly due to the fact that they are rich in antioxidants, which offer an important defence against atherosclerosis (and against cancer). The 'ACE' antioxidants are beta-carotene (a form of Vitamin A), Vitamin C and Vitamin E. Together with another important antioxidant, selenium, these 'ACE' heart-health agents are found in a whole range of fruits, vegetables and nuts.

Another benefit of fruit and vegetables is that they provide a good source of potassium, which may help to control blood pressure, and folic acid, which may help to reduce the level of homocysteine, another risk factor in heart disease. It is best to eat a wide range of fruit and vegetables – and these can be fresh, frozen, dried or tinned. (Note that potatoes don't count as a vegetable for the 'Five-a-day' advice, but instead are considered to be a starchy food.) One portion will look something like the size of a clenched fist, and five portions will weigh around 500 g (just over 1 lb). You can also try eating fruit and vegetables that reflect the colours of a rainbow – red (e.g. red peppers, tomatoes, watermelon), orange (e.g. carrots, oranges, sweet potatoes), yellow (e.g. bananas, sweetcorn, pineapples), green (e.g. broccoli, cabbage, watercress), blue (e.g. blueberries, blackberries, prunes), indigo/violet (e.g. aubergines, beetroot, plums). Eating a variety of such fruit and vegetables will help to protect us from heart disease and stroke, and the Stroke Association (see page 120) counsels us to 'Eat a rainbow, beat a stroke'.

- *Cut down on saturated fats and replace them with moderate amounts of unsaturated fats*

A high saturated-fat intake can result in raising cholesterol levels, so saturates should be limited in a heart-healthy diet. All the fats we encounter in food are a mixture of saturates, polyunsaturates and monounsaturates. Some foods may also include trans-fatty acids (trans-fats) which are produced by a process called hydrogenation – used to turn unsaturated vegetable oils into solid fat, as in margarine. Trans-fats act like saturates, increasing total cholesterol levels.

Monounsaturated and polyunsaturated fats, on the other hand, help to keep cholesterol levels down, as do spreads (or foods) fortified with plant stanols or sterols. Polyunsaturated fats also tend to reduce blood stickiness, and can help to protect the heart from arrhythmias (abnormal heart rhythms). Examples of foods that contain monounsaturated fats are: olive and rapeseed oil, peanut oil, several margarines and spreads, and avocados. Polyunsaturated fats, on the other hand, can be found in sunflower oils, some nut oils, many margarines and spreads, walnuts, pumpkins, and leafy vegetables such as spinach.

Saturates (the fats to limit) are contained in fatty meats, whole milk, cream, hard cheese, butter, and they are also present as 'hidden fats' in lots of biscuits, cakes, pastries and take-away foods. For most situations, we would recommend the use of unsaturated oils or margarine, rather than hard margarines and butter, which are high in saturates. Olive or rapeseed oil, for example, can have particularly beneficial effects on blood lipid levels, but other unsaturated oils are also fine for cooking.

- *Reduce the total amount of fat you eat – especially if you are overweight*

Although, as we have seen, not all fats are 'bad', fats *are* nevertheless rich in calories, and a high fat intake is likely to lead to an excess in weight – unless, of course, you take a lot of exercise to burn it off. One thing that is clear is that if your energy intake is greater than your energy expenditure, you will certainly put on weight. In *Eating for a Healthy Heart*, a 'Traffic Light' system is provided to help you to work out how much fat is a reasonable amount in any one portion of food. In general terms:

10 g or less fat per portion   represents   **GREEN for GO**
(with saturated fat closer to
1 g than 5 g)

20 g or more fat   represents   **RED for STOP**
(and 5 g or more saturated)

- *Aim to eat at least one serving of oily fish each week*

Oily fish contains omega-3 polyunsaturated fatty acids, which have been found to help prevent potentially fatal heart arrhythmias and thrombosis (blood clots). They also lower triglyceride levels (see page 12) and may help to lower blood pressure and increase the 'good' HDL cholesterol. Oily fish include herrings, mackerel, kippers, sardines, salmon, trout and fresh tuna.

At the time of writing, the guidelines suggest that most people should aim to eat two portions of fish a week, *one* of which is oily; but if you have recently had a heart attack, there may be some extra benefit in eating up to *three* portions of oily fish a week (or fish capsules to provide between 500 mg and 1000 mg of omega-3 fat per day).

- *Keep to a healthy weight (if you are overweight, try to lose some weight – especially around your waist)*

Keeping a healthy weight for your height will help to keep your blood pressure under control, and reduce the workload for your heart. One way of checking whether you are overweight is to use a BMI (Body Mass Index) chart (see page 82). When you go for a check-up, your doctor will probably use this chart to confirm that you are not overweight, and you can use the Index, as we have suggested, to keep an eye on your weight. (Another measure that is sometimes used in assessing risk for cardiovascular disease and diabetes is waist circumference. At the time of writing, there is still some controversy over this measure, especially in relation to the selection of appropriate cut-off points, but it has been suggested that, in very general terms, a waist measurement above 102 cm/40 in for a man, or 88 cm/35 in for a woman, tends to indicate an increased level of risk.)

• *Reduce the portion size of food you eat*

Often we can stop ourselves from becoming overweight by simply reducing the size of the portions we eat. This is probably the simplest (and possibly the most effective) piece of advice we can offer if you are concerned that you tend to become overweight easily.

• *Cut down on salt*

The sodium contained in salt has been found to be linked to high blood pressure which, as we have already seen, is one of the most important risk factors for heart disease and stroke. The recommended *daily* intake of salt from all sources is below 7 g for men and 5 g for women. Much of your daily intake will come from the 'hidden' salt found in processed foods and bread, so the best advice is to try to avoid using any additional salt, and start checking food labels! If you look at the information giving the amount of sodium and salt per 100 g portion, the general 'healthy eating' guidelines at the time of writing are that 0.6 g sodium is 'a lot' and 0.1 g 'a little'; and for salt 1.5 g is 'a lot' and 0.3 g 'a little'.

• *Eat cholesterol-lowering foods*

A number of foods (in addition to unsaturated oils) can help to control cholesterol levels. Fruit and vegetables, pulses such as beans, peas, lentils and chickpeas, and oats, all contain gums, gels or pectin, which help to reduce blood cholesterol levels, and slow down the rate at which sugar is released into the bloodstream. The antioxidants in fruit and vegetables help to reduce the build-up of cholesterol deposits in our arteries (see page 84), and flavonoids and phenols (the antioxidant compounds that give fruit and vegetables their colour) are also present in wine (especially red wine), grape juice, tea and in chocolate (especially dark chocolate). So, in moderation, both alcohol and chocolate can have beneficial effects. Garlic is also considered by many to be a valuable cholesterol-lowering food.

• *Try to choose items of food that are low on the Glycaemic Index (GI)*

The Glycaemic Index (GI) shows how foods affect blood glucose levels, and those with a *low* index provide a slow and sustained release of glucose. They also increase levels of the 'good' HDL cholesterol, help to prevent the furring up of arteries, and generally reduce our risk of developing or exacerbating diabetes and heart problems. Here are some examples of foods with a low GI index: oats and bran, lentils, pasta, basmati rice and couscous, beans of all kinds (but soya and kidney beans are especially low), multi-grain/ wholegrain breads, skimmed milk, low-fat yogurt, fruits like apples, oranges, grapefruit, apricots, pears, peaches, plums and cherries. (See also Glycaemic Index website, address on page 120.)

• *Drink alcohol within sensible limits*

Moderate drinking (between 1 and 2 units per day) can be heart-protective. However, heavier drinking can contribute to disorders of the heart muscle, high blood pressure, and stroke. Men are recommended to drink no more than 4 units per day (and 21 units per week), whereas women are recommended to drink no more than 3 units per day (and 14 units per week). A unit is half a pint of beer, a single 25-ml measure of spirits, or a small (125-ml) glass of wine. It is also recommended that you have two alcohol-free days per week.

Common queries about healthy eating

Below we offer a few suggestions for dealing with common queries about healthy eating.

I already eat a healthy diet; do I really need to change it?

First, are you *sure* you have a healthy diet? Despite the information provided on food labels, it is still quite difficult to keep a check on the nutritional value of the food we eat, especially if much of it is processed. When people start to analyse their food intake (e.g. by keeping a 'food diary', as we suggest below) they are often surprised at what it contains! Also, if you are overweight, or are putting on weight, there is a strong probability that you are eating a greater amount than is required for the energy that your body expends. Even if you are not overweight, you may still not be eating as healthily as you could, and in some cases you might even be eating some foods that are distinctly 'unfriendly' to your heart.

Research shows us that one of the reasons why people do not tend to change to eating healthier diets is because they believe that they are already eating healthily, when in fact they are not. It is only by using computer packages that calculate the constituents of the amount and type of foods you eat, that a true representation of your nutrient intake can be given. However, in the real world, this is rarely possible, so we have to use proxy measures instead to estimate the healthiness of our diets. A good place to start is to write down everything that you eat and drink for a week (a kind of food and drink diary), so that you can clearly see the range and amount of food you are eating. Be honest with yourself and make sure that you write down the type and amounts of foods and drinks you have eaten for each meal – and don't forget the mid-morning snacks! It may also be helpful to write down the times and situations when you eat (both snacks and main meals), so that you can see whether certain things seem to trigger a snacking habit, for example. Once you have done this for a week, there are a number of things you can check for:

- Did you eat five portions of fruit and vegetables per day?
- Are you eating a good variety of fruit and vegetables?
- Did you eat a portion of oily fish?
- Are the foods you eat mostly low on the Glycaemic Index?

If you have answered 'no' to any of these questions, then you can take steps to improve your diet. Now here are some more to check:

- How many food portions did you eat that contained 'a lot' of fat?
- How many food portions did you eat that contained 'a lot' of *saturated* fat?
- How many times did you fry, rather than grill or bake food?
- How many items did you eat that contained salt?
- How much alcohol did you drink in total?
- How many times did you snack on biscuits or chocolate bars?

If the items containing saturated fat or salt are looking rather high, or if you have fried food more often than grilled, then you might want to consider changing your diet to include healthier alternatives. It would also be useful to add up your alcohol 'units' – did you manage to drink sensibly, or were you drinking more than the recommendations suggest? Were you drinking a glass of wine over a leisurely meal with food (the recommended approach to taking on alcoholic beverages – see section on the Mediterranean diet below) or were you 'binge-drinking' alcohol (the worst conceivable approach to drinking)? If you found you tended to snack on biscuits or chocolate bars, try substituting a bit of carrot, fruit or nuts instead. If you have the opportunity, you may find it useful to discuss this food diary with a dietitian, or practice nurse, who should be able to help you to think about ways in which you can improve it.

I've heard people recommending the Mediterranean diet. What is this?

People living in Mediterranean countries (like the southern parts of France and Italy, and Greece) have some of the lowest rates of coronary heart disease. It is widely believed that one of the factors contributing to their good heart-health is diet. So why not go Mediterranean!

Here are some of the features of the Mediterranean diet:

- Plenty of fresh fruit and vegetables, pulses and beans, bread, pasta, rice and salads.
- Unprocessed, home-cooked food that is grilled, steamed or baked, or lightly cooked in oil high in a monounsaturated fat, such as olive oil, with lots of herbs.
- Plenty of both white and oily fish, and small quantities of lean meat.
- Food eaten at a leisurely pace, with wine (especially red) to accompany the meal.

Aren't healthy diets a lot of work, boring and expensive?

Healthy eating doesn't have to be boring; there are now many cookery books containing tasty recipes specifically aimed towards healthy eating. If you are not interested in cooking for yourself, or don't have much time, most supermarkets now provide a range of healthy, low-fat meals. Heart-healthy eating might mean a change in the foods that you buy and eat. Make any changes gradually, and regard it as an opportunity to try new foods, rather than a chore. The belief that healthy eating is expensive puts many people off changing to a healthier diet. However, there is little evidence to support this view – in fact, eating a heavily meat-based diet with a high fat content, for example, is considerably more expensive than eating a low-fat vegetarian diet.

How do I decide which changes to make?

Once you have decided that your diet requires modifying, the next step is to decide which changes you need or want to make. Here are some suggestions that might help:

- Swap your full-fat milk for semi-skimmed (or semi-skimmed for skimmed milk).
- Try grilling rather than frying food.
- If you eat red meat, trim off the visible fat.
- If you eat chicken, make sure you take off the skin.
- When you eat cooked vegetables or potatoes, steam rather than boil to help retain the nutrients, and don't add butter or margarine.
- Avoid creamy dressings on salads; either give the dressing a miss or use low-fat dressing.
- Cut down on your portion sizes (especially if you are overweight).
- Eat fruit, carrots or nuts rather than biscuits as a mid-morning snack.
- Inspect the labels of food you buy in the supermarket, and check for fat and salt content.
- Remove salt from your table – don't add extra salt to food.
- Cut down on your alcohol intake.

It is important that you make the changes gradually, rather than making any drastic modifications to your diet. Pick a couple of things you want to work on, and go from there. Try and think ahead to any obstacles that you might come across, and plan ways of getting around them. If you can't decide which changes to make first, write a list and then prioritize them in terms of which ones are likely to provide most benefit.

I've decided which changes I'm going to make, but how do I go about making them?

Treat the changes as an experiment. Decide when, where and how you are going to make the changes, and then go for it! You might find it helps if you write down the changes you are targeting on a bit of paper and then stick it in a prominent place, such as the fridge door. Some people find it useful to have an overall goal to motivate them – for example, reducing weight to 70 kg (11 stone), or being able to go up a particular flight of stairs without getting out of breath. If you have such a goal in mind, you need to make sure first of all that it is achievable (i.e. don't try to lose enough weight to fit into four shirt sizes below your current size in a week!). If it is *not* achievable, set a new goal that is more realistic and make the changes slowly and gradually, taking one step at a time.

If you can encourage someone else to make the changes with you, this might also help. Try to maintain the changes for a week or two, so that you have a chance to get used to them, and to give your palate time to adapt to the new tastes – you never know, you might even find that you don't want to go back to your old diet anyway!

I've had a go, and failed. What shall I do now?

If you treat the changes as an experiment, then you need to remember that these experiments don't really 'pass' or 'fail'. You have set one up to see how you get on and to note the results. An experiment that has not worked is as important as one that has, and you can still learn a lot from it. Write down any obstacles that have come up along the way, and start thinking of different ways to get around them. You might also find it helpful to discuss them with your practice nurse, dietitian, or friend/partner who has made the changes with you. For example:

Obstacle: 'I did not stick to my diet when I was invited to Sarah's house for a meal. I just ate what was put on the plate in front of me.'
Solution: 'Next time I'll phone Sarah ahead of the meal and discuss some examples of what might be "on" or "off" the menu for me. Although this may feel awkward, it's likely that Sarah will understand and it will be much less awkward to pre-warn her ahead of time than if I arrive and I can't eat anything on the menu again.'

Finally, it is also important that if you *do* give in to that extra glass of wine or piece of cake occasionally, don't punish yourself and consider yourself a failure, but instead view it as a 'one off' and continue with your healthy eating plan as usual. We're all allowed the occasional treat!

I'm finding it difficult to stick to the changes. What can I do about it?

Making the initial changes to your diet is one big step in the right direction. However, if you want to see the long-term benefits of eating healthily, you will need to make sure that you stick to the changes you have made. Eventually, you will not even have to think about the changes because they will start becoming part of your normal routine. However, until then it is important that you persevere with them. Many people find this the tricky bit, and it is at this point that they end up giving in and returning to their previous dietary habits.

If you find yourself 'giving in' more often than not, one tip is to try and think about the reasons why. Is it because you were feeling stressed, anxious or fed up? Or were you feeling happy, energetic and full of life? If you do find a link between lapses in your diet and the way you were feeling at the time, here is a technique you could use:

If you find yourself feeling fed up and about to buy yourself chocolate bars or alcoholic drinks for comfort, try to imagine how you would feel after you have consumed them. Happy and less fed up? Or do you think that you would feel regret, less healthy and *more* fed up? Sometimes this technique can be quite effective, and can stop you from giving in when you are feeling low. People who turn to food or drink for comfort often feel considerably worse after they have binged, rather than better.

A final tip is to keep reminding yourself of the reasons why you have made these changes. Remind yourself of all the *negative* things associated with going back to your old diet – you might find it useful to write these down and put them in prominent places around the house. Then remind yourself of all the *positive* things that can be gained from eating healthily. What is the evidence? If you find it difficult to remember, have a look at the first part of the chapter again to jog your memory!

13

Strategies for self-managing your health

Self-management of health is something that we generally take for granted when we are well, treating minor ailments by tried and trusted methods such as taking an aspirin and sitting down quietly if we feel a migraine coming on, using a cream to treat hard or dry skin, or buying over-the-counter remedies to relieve the symptoms of a stuffy cold. However, some people are happy to handle minor problems, but lack confidence when it comes to managing health issues that may have more serious consequences than the odd cough or cold. Or they may be used to placing all their trust and reliance in doctors to monitor their health. Others may have an internal need to be in control of those decisions and care procedures that can impact so directly on their health.

Whichever type of person you perceive yourself to be, whether a passive recipient of healthcare, or a keen partner in the treatment process, it is helpful to acknowledge that your physical and emotional progress during rehabilitation is at least partly dependent on your *own* thoughts, feelings and actions, and this is where some knowledge of self-management strategies is useful. This chapter offers you some suggestions on general issues, and in the next chapter we concentrate specifically on managing stress.

Check that your knowledge and beliefs about your condition are sound

One of the most important aspects of health self-management is the need to make sure that you have a sound understanding of your condition and how best to keep yourself in good health after your bypass. For example, it will be helpful to know about the factors associated with keeping your heart healthy, how medication helps, and why your rehabilitation programme is important (see Chapters 3, 5 and 10). Sometimes people misunderstand the reasons for certain pieces of advice. If they are told that they should 'take it easy' after the bypass, for example, this might be misinterpreted as meaning 'avoid physical exercise after your bypass'. As we have seen, however, taking regular physical exercise is, in fact, an essential part of the rehabilitation process. The advice to 'take it easy' is a warning not to engage in over-strenuous exercise, rather than avoid exercise altogether!

Carry out frequent reality checks on your beliefs

Living with a cardiac condition means that you will have developed a set of beliefs about your experiences. These may not always represent sound beliefs and they may require revision as you gain more knowledge and experience about your condition and its treatment. So it's important that you carry out frequent reality checks on your beliefs to make sure that you have modified them to take account of information and advice you have been given, or have obtained from your own experiences. This is important because our beliefs have a direct bearing on the way we perceive information and events, and help to determine what sort of actions we are willing to take.

For example, while his health was relatively good, Stephen (page 32) clung to the belief that giving up smoking wasn't absolutely essential. He tried to quit, but soon slipped back into his old habits. However, doing a reality check when he was diagnosed with diabetes changed all that. He knew diabetes was a major risk factor for heart disease and that smoking added substantially to this risk. Persuaded by this reality check, he set about putting his new beliefs into action. On this occasion, he quit smoking permanently within a few months. Despite the damage that had already been done to his coronary arteries, stopping smoking improved his general health, aided his recovery from bypass surgery, and helped to reduce his risk of developing further heart problems later on.

Establish your own benchmarks for recognizing problem symptoms

One of the common questions that people ask after surgery is, 'How will I know if there is something wrong or if I am getting worse?' Try to establish some sort of 'symptom benchmark' by which you can assess the severity of the symptoms you are experiencing. This is partly a function of time, of course, and there is an understandable tendency in the early days after the operation to interpret certain pains as indicative of heart problems when they are, in fact, unrelated to the heart. After a while, however, you will become quite expert at discriminating different sorts of pain. For example, most people find that they are soon able to discriminate physical symptoms related to heart problems from those related to post-operative physical sensations (e.g. wound pain). Similarly, a spot of indigestion can often be recognized as such (rather than angina) by ascertaining that it is remedied by an indigestion tablet rather than a nitrate spray! Establishing these benchmarks will help you to self-manage your health with increasing confidence.

Set yourself specific goals

We have already discussed the value of setting goals or targets in the initial phase of recovery (see page 64), but this continues to be important all the way through your rehabilitation and is a crucial part of health self-management. Once past the immediate post-surgery period, when you are increasing your physical capabilities, you will feel able to take on tasks, jobs or roles that you held prior to surgery. However, when identifying your goals you will need to have specific and precise thoughts about the outcomes. For example, David (page 64) might have set himself a *vague* goal by saying to himself: 'I will walk a bit further tomorrow'; whereas what he did, in fact, was to set himself a *specific* goal (always the most effective strategy) – in his case, to reach a particular tree or lamp post that was farther than one he reached on an earlier walk.

It can be helpful to divide some activities into sub-goals so that you can build up the overall performance gradually, starting with sub-goals that are realistic and achievable in relation to your current level of fitness. With this in mind, it's worth sometimes asking: 'Am I trying to jump too far ahead?' If you think this is the case, then try fewer, shorter or less intensive steps (or sub-goals) first in order to allow your body and mind a chance to readjust and work towards the larger goal.

Robert, for example, set as one of his targets 'to get back to skiing' (see page 76) and, with the help of the physios in his rehab class, he broke down this overall target into sub-goals. His first task was to get his body into reasonable physical shape after the bypass, and he accomplished this by working hard on his rehab course. Then the rehab physios provided a specific programme to help get the 'skiing muscles' warmed up, and Robert carried on with this after his rehab had finished: 'doing exercises in the gym to tone me up for this – three times a week in the gym'. His next sub-goal, several months down the line, was to check out his progress by practising on a dry-ski slope, and finally he made it back to skiing in Switzerland within a year of his bypass.

This measured approach is certainly worth trying if you are finding temporarily that some of your overall goals appear a little out of range in the early recovery period.

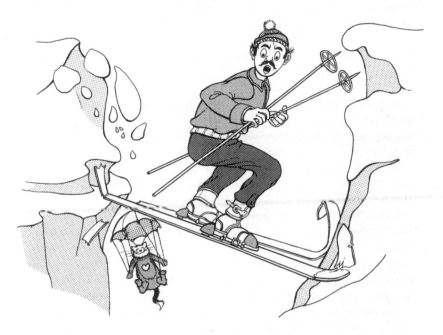

Trying to jump too far . . .

Pace your activities

This approach to achieving goals in a realistic manner is termed 'pacing'. It has been shown to be a helpful strategy for people undergoing rehabilitation for various forms of surgery and particularly for cardiac problems. The staff leading your cardiac rehabilitation programme will also advocate this method and will support and advise you. However, it is important that you carry over this approach to your home-based goals throughout rehabilitation.

A common concern is people's ability to identify safe boundaries surrounding home activity and exercise – this is the question 'How do I know if I'm doing too much?' We have already examined appropriate exercise levels in Chapter 11 in the context of a supervised rehab programme, but if you are posing this question later on during your self-management stage, then it's probably due to the feeling that you're able to do more than you are doing already, or that you are trying out activities (e.g. mowing the lawn or doing weekly shopping trips to the supermarket) and are unsure about the potential impact these activities might have on you. Remember that the leaflets and information you are given after bypass surgery cover general aspects of rehabilitation and do not cover all aspects of your particular lifestyle, roles, responsibilities and activities. So there will be tasks or activities that you will want, and feel able, to undertake that may not have been discussed by your rehab team or GP. You will be able to assess your readiness to take on such activities by breaking down the sub-elements of the task, as we have described above, and checking these yourself before you engage in the full task.

But it's important that you don't take physical risks with your recovering body, and there will be some tasks for which it would be sensible to obtain professional advice before engaging in them. For example, putting direct questions to professionals about tasks that involve heavy lifting and manual handling or prolonged intensive exercise is vital.

In particular, if you fail to pace yourself adequately, then you will have more difficulty maximizing the self-belief and confidence that are so essential to maintaining the successful self-management of your post-bypass health. You can then become trapped in a 'vicious circle' in which worrying about an activity leads to a reduction or avoidance in its performance and a consequent decrease in confidence in the ability to perform the activity, and so back to increased worry again. If this vicious circle is not broken, then confidence will spiral downwards and negatively impact on your progress.

A simple illustration of how to prevent the vicious circle developing is provided by Sheila (whose case is described in Chapter 14). She stayed with her daughter in London after her op and both of them were worried about Sheila going out for a walk in a busy London street: 'The first day we went out for a walk my daughter was really frightened that someone might knock into me or something. So we worked out the quietest time of the day for our little walk.' Sheila could easily have simply stayed indoors and avoided the activity, but this would then have started the vicious circle already described. Her confidence about going out for a walk would have tended to decrease, and her worry about coping outdoors would have become even more intense, making her goal of going out for a walk even less easy to achieve. However, Sheila was determined that her fear was not going to stop her progress. So she 'tested the water', with her daughter as a walking companion and back-up 'nurse'! These short walks gave her the concrete experience she needed to check on the achievability of her goal. She paced herself well, going for a gentle stroll to begin with when the streets were quiet, and gradually building up to walking independently to the local shops. Sheila rewarded herself with a cup of tea and one of her daughter's home-baked scones when she got back in!

Stephen (Chapter 5) explains his way of defeating the vicious circle: 'Don't just sit around feeling sorry for yourself and letting your partner do all the running around. It can be a bit scary at first because you think you've got to be careful about doing too much. But doing too *little* and letting your anxiety about your heart problems rule your life is much worse in the end. Work at increasing your exercise levels steadily, and take advantage of any rehabilitation sessions you're offered and you'll find that your confidence will quickly return, and you'll be 100 per cent fitter than you were before. That's what I've found, anyway.'

If you hadn't developed the skills of health self-management before your bypass, you will soon find that you will discover your own ways of coping during your rehabilitation. Piecing your life back together during this period is a bit like doing a jigsaw puzzle. Some pieces of your life will start to fit together again quickly and easily, whereas others may only start to slot in later on when you can see the pattern of your new post-bypass life emerging more clearly. But by then you will be well on your way to getting back to work and/or home routines and restoring a much better quality of life than you had been experiencing before your bypass.

Before we look at this long-anticipated part of the journey, however, we examine in the next chapter some specific suggestions about how you can best help yourself to cope with stress.

14
Coping with stress

During rehabilitation you will have been given advice about modifying risk factors for further cardiac problems, including eating a healthier diet, taking more exercise and controlling your weight, blood pressure and cholesterol. But 'stress management' may also have been mentioned, and learning how to cope effectively with stress can greatly benefit your recovery.

In Chapter 3 we described the physiological changes that take place when our bodies are faced with danger – the 'fight or flight' reaction. These changes are associated with symptoms such as a dry mouth, trembling hands and voice, wobbly knees, or a 'tight band' around the forehead. When the danger recedes, the body returns to normal and these feelings go away.

A certain amount of stress is valuable, of course, as a sort of energizer which spurs us on to get things done. The problems for most people tend to arise, however, when the level of stress remains at a constant high, usually because the threats do not arise from temporary physical dangers but from other situations that we perceive as stressful, such as pressures at work or difficult interpersonal relationships. These situations are often more pervasive and less susceptible to swift resolution than occasional physical threats. In these circumstances the body prepares for 'flight or fight' and remains in a state of constant alert rather than calming down after the threat has been dealt with. Then blood pressure and heart rate tend to remain too high, the blood's tendency to clot increases, and the level of protective HDL cholesterol is reduced – all features that represent cardiovascular risk factors and that are harmful to good heart-health.

Recognizing stress in your life

It is advisable, therefore, to try to recognize any negative stressors in your daily life and to modify them. As we have seen (page 14), people who exhibit traits such as aggression, competitiveness, anger and hostility are particularly at risk of having unhealthy stress levels. But whatever type of person you are, it's a good idea to try to identify the triggers that increase your stress levels by looking at both external factors (e.g. the tendency to react to other people's comments or behaviour by getting into highly emotive arguments with them) and internal ones (e.g. personal worries). It can be useful to note down situations in which you find that you become stressed, and to monitor the thought processes, emotions and physiological sensations that you experience on such occasions. Writing them down often helps to clarify the factors contributing to the stress, e.g. when they occur most frequently, what sort of events tend to precipitate their occurrence, and what sort of reactions you experience. Then you can set about trying to modify them.

For example, imagine that you had jotted down the occasions on which you became stressed and found that most of them related to being late for appointments. One of the main triggers for stress in this case might be poor time management, leaving too little time to get to appointments. Your notes might read something like this:

Situation: Stuck in a traffic jam in the car. Late for an important meeting with X and Y.
Thoughts: 'It will look to X and Y as if I don't think our meeting is important', 'They won't believe I was in a jam', 'What stupidity has caused this jam?', 'How can I get out of this quicker?' 'Idiots blocking the road!'
Emotional responses: Angry, frustrated and anxious.
Behavioural: Shouting and shaking fist at windscreen, winding windows up and down.
Physiological responses: Headache, heart pounding, twinges of chest pain, feeling nauseous.

Thoughts, emotions, behaviours and physical sensations all combine to produce your specific stress responses and you will often find that your reactions are based on negative (and sometimes irrational) views. Your task is to aim to replace these negative thoughts by more useful, positive ones. You can use a process called 'self-talk' to help you do this, reflecting to yourself the thoughts that you were having during the stressful events and replacing them with more positive (and rational) ones. To begin with, you need to check the accuracy and validity of your thoughts so that you can challenge them on a rational basis. (For more help with this sort of approach, see *Stress at Work* by Mary Hartley, full details on page 120.) With regard to being late, for example:

Thoughts: 'X and Y know me better than that – they know how much I value our meetings', 'I can't do anything to get there quicker, but I must make sure I leave more time in future', 'We can re-schedule the meeting', 'I can pull off the road and phone in to explain', 'No harm done'.

Emotional responses: Resignation, calm.

Behavioural: Relax in seat, open window to allow in more air (not to shout at another driver!) and to aid relaxation and deeper breathing, listen to radio.

Physiological responses: More stable, less arousal as a result of positive thoughts and actions.

Here are a few other suggestions for keeping stress levels in hand:

- Prioritize the demands on your time, so that you don't try to do too many things – start by writing a list of 'things to do' and then rearrange them in order of priority.
- Don't worry about saying 'no' to people if you feel something would be too much for you – just explain that you don't feel up to it at present.
- Pace yourself so that you don't ask your body to cope with too much physical or mental activity.
- A pet such as a dog or a cat can help to keep your stress levels down and speed your recovery after your bypass.
- Learn how to relax and try some of the relaxation exercises we describe below.

Relaxation techniques

Relaxation techniques can provide excellent skills with which to combat stress and, applied on an everyday basis, will lower the average level of cardiovascular response to stress (called cardiovascular reactivity) and reduce long-term cardiovascular risks. It is necessary to practise deep relaxation in non-stressful conditions first, so that it is easier to learn to apply the techniques during times of increased stress. Practising relaxation takes time (like any skill) and requires regular sessions of about 20 minutes per day until you are familiar with the exercises.

Progressive muscular relaxation comprises the repeated tensing and relaxing of muscle groups throughout the body, from your toes up to your head, in a systematic way. Sometimes called 'deep relaxation', this can either be learned through your cardiac rehab programme or self-taught following pre-recorded relaxation tapes (see page 120). If you choose to use the tapes or CDs, then pick a time of day when you know you will not be interrupted, and one that is not too near to your bedtime (otherwise it is being used as a sleep-aid rather than a stress-busting skill).

Recognizing physical tension in your muscles and learning how to reduce it in a scenario that is not pressurized will be useful for identifying such tensions in more stressful situations. Once you have established this process through deep relaxation, you can move on to identifying triggers for tension or stress, as already described, and then practise relaxation in response to them.

You can also help to keep your general levels of tension as low as possible by practising relaxation at different times during the day (not just in response to trigger points). For example, you could identify certain times, such as tea/coffee breaks, and use these to remind yourself to do a few relaxation exercises. By doing this regularly you will be helping to control your stress levels and reducing the concomitant effects on your cardiovascular system.

Dealing with panic attacks

During rehab, some people go through short periods of emotions such as feelings of anxiety and even the occasional panic attack (panic is not exclusive to people with cardiac problems, of course). Some people may have one or two panic attacks shortly after they return home from hospital; others may have them over a longer period. They are quite common: *not* a sign of a serious emotional or physical illness, and *not* dangerous. However, if these panic attacks are not dealt with quickly, then they can affect your mood and cause you to feel low, unmotivated or fearful. These feelings can develop when people assume that panic is something that they have to put up with or live with. You should certainly not assume that this is the case since there are strategies to manage it. We discuss some of these below.

Recognizing and understanding panic
Panic symptoms are nothing more than an extreme form of fear, and a panic attack is a strong feeling of terror that comes on very suddenly. Physical symptoms include a pounding heart, fast breathing (also called hyperventilation), shaking, wobbly legs – all caused

by the increased surge of adrenaline in your body. Other feelings can include a sense of unreality and increased anxiety. People often have frightening thoughts (e.g. 'I'm going to die' or 'I'm losing control') and think something awful is happening. The feelings often seem to come suddenly, 'like a wave'. But although it is disturbing, panic in itself is not dangerous or harmful.

Panic attacks can occur when there is no obvious physical threat. For people recovering from cardiac surgery, however, they generally tend to occur when associations are made mistakenly between physical sensations related to surgical recovery (e.g. wound pain in the chest) and cardiac symptoms such as angina, or when real physical symptoms are perceived as life-threatening (but are not). Often people with cardiac symptoms who experience panic will find it difficult to discriminate between actual symptoms and panic sensations, and they may attribute panic sensations to a worsening of their physical condition. For example, they might assume that a pounding heart indicates a heart problem, when there are, in fact, no cardiac rhythm problems.

If you start to feel panicky, try jotting down your thoughts and feelings in a diary, as suggested earlier for dealing with stress (see page 101). This will help you to identify the sorts of situations in which you tend to feel panicky, what seems to trigger it, what your thoughts are when you are experiencing panic, and how you tend to deal with these feelings. You will then be able to find ways of reacting to the panic attacks in a more rational way.

Steps in managing panic

- *Accept that panic cannot harm you.* This is a crucial element in dealing with it.
- *Slow down your breathing.* During a panic attack people often hyperventilate and breathe out too much carbon dioxide. This can make you feel dizzy or give you feelings of 'pins and needles'.
- *Keep a paper bag handy* to help improve the balance of carbon dioxide if you hyperventilate. Breathe into the bag slowly and then re-breathe the air. Repeat this up to ten times and then remove the bag and breathe normally again. Repeat the process as necessary.
- *Stop focusing on your body.* Focus instead on what is going on outside rather than inside you.
- *Distract yourself from frightening thoughts.* You need to do this

for about three minutes to reduce symptoms. For example, listen very carefully to someone talking, or think of a favourite scene in your mind. Try singing a song to yourself or type a mobile phone text message. Really concentrate.

- *Question and test your frightening thoughts.* Although distraction is good in the short term, in the long run it is most helpful to challenge your thoughts, so that you no longer believe them. Check your 'panic diary' and ask yourself: 'What is the evidence for and against my worries? How many times have I had these thoughts and has my worst fear ever happened?'
- *Don't worry if the panic attacks don't stop immediately.* Instead, check in your 'panic diary' and remind yourself that nothing terrible actually does happen as a result of a panic attack.
- *Try to ease your way back into situations that seem to trigger panic attacks.* Test yourself by entering such a situation briefly, and then removing yourself from it and giving yourself a reward of some kind. For example, if you tend to panic while doing a week's shopping in the supermarket, just pop into the shop, buy one item as a reward and leave; then gradually build up the length of exposure to the supermarket until you can cope with a basketful of shopping, and so on.
- *Take a friend with you for support.* If you need to build up your confidence in coping with certain situations, take a friend with you for support, or get in touch with staff on your rehab course. Rehab courses differ in the facilities they can offer, but many will be only too willing to help. As one course co-ordinator puts it: 'People can be referred into our counselling service at any point in time, and they can also refer themselves. Sometimes we have people who go all the way through rehab and they finish; and they ring me up a month later and say, "I've suddenly started getting panic attacks. Can I see somebody?" And in these circumstances we'll always try to help.' It's certainly much better to confront the panic situations rather than to avoid them, since avoidance will tend to reduce the extent of your confidence in your approach to health self-management.

Stress can also rear its destructive head in the context of family life, partly as a result of the extra burdens and anxieties that are placed on other family members during both the pre- and post-bypass experience. (We look more fully at how bypass surgery affects the family in the next chapter.)

Sheila

Sheila is in her mid-sixties, a divorced mother of four grown-up children, a boy and a three girls. For many years she was a senior manager in a residential home for people with learning difficulties. She still needed to pay off the mortgage, so she carried on working after she had reached retirement age. But she found she got so stressed and felt so tired that she left this job and took another (less pressurized) post as a care worker: 'I just thought the tiredness was because I had such a stressful job and I was getting older.'

She liked her new less stressful job but her tiredness persisted, and one day she experienced some chest pains that caused her considerable alarm. She was coming back from town, carrying several bags of shopping. She got off the bus and, while walking the few hundred yards to her home, she developed severe pains in her chest. These pains were so strong that she had to stop several times before she got home.

Sheila knew that she had a number of cardiovascular risk factors. Apart from a family history of heart disease (her father had suffered from angina and died from a heart attack at the age of 71), she had been under stress at work, was overweight, and suffered from high blood pressure.

She recognized the pains as similar to those her father used to get and her GP confirmed her own suspicions: that she was probably suffering from angina. He gave her a nitrate spray and told her to carry on with her life as usual. If she found the pain coming on, then she should use the spray.

The first time she had to use the spray was when she was on her way to see her GP for a follow-up visit. The pain suddenly started to spread across her chest and in her back, so she used the spray and found that it worked. She was pleased that the pain went off, but she was also upset because she felt that this definitely showed that the pain was angina – and this meant that, like her father, she *did* have heart problems. Her GP agreed with this diagnosis and thought it was time he referred her to a cardiologist.

Because of the long waiting period for cardiology appointments, Sheila decided to book an appointment privately. She wanted to get things sorted out as soon as possible. She used to look after her two youngest grandchildren who at that time were three and one, and she thought, 'My God, supposing something really awful happened and I'm looking after them – and I died on them! I can't wait and wait for an appointment.'

The cardiologist checked out her cholesterol level, which was raised (about 7.0 mmol/L), and arranged to give her a stress ECG as well as the normal resting version: 'I had to go on the treadmill, but I couldn't even do two minutes on that!' The stress ECG indicated pronounced heart problems, and the cardiologist referred her for an immediate angiogram, which revealed two badly furred-up arteries for which she would need a bypass operation.

'I was so upset. Really, really shocked. I just thought he was going to say, "You're going to need tablets" – because I swim, I cycle, I walk, I don't smoke . . . But the cardiologist said if I don't have it, my chances of having a heart attack were very great . . . so I said, "What are my chances of surviving this op?" and he said, "You've got a 99 per cent chance". So I thought, well, that's better than the odds of having a heart attack.' Sheila also asked the consultant about flying to see her daughter in the USA: 'He wouldn't let me fly before the op. He said, "You can't, you'll die – you'll have a heart attack up there",.'

The cardiologist also reviewed Sheila's medication. He put her on 40 mg simvastatin to lower her cholesterol, and he added 50 mg atenolol as an anti-angina drug which would also help to bring down her blood pressure. He asked her to continue with her existing anti-hypertension medication (40 mg lisinopril a day), and with the daily 75 mg dose of aspirin. Then five days before the op, she was told to stop all her medication.

Although she went for a private consultation with the cardiologist, Sheila decided she couldn't afford to have the operation done privately, and had to wait five months for her bypass: 'The surgeon asked me, "What do you want to do if we do this op?" And I said, "Well, I really would like to be able to run again 'cos I can't run and I can't take the grandchildren anywhere." We had to stay in 'cos I was so frightened if they ran off. I couldn't catch them. I'd given up swimming. If I went swimming in the sea, my brother and sister-in-law came with me . . . they knew where my spray was . . . Well, if I went by myself, who would know if I was waving or drowning from a heart attack! . . . I thought if I have the bypass and I can do all these things again, then it's worth it.'

When Sheila was admitted to hospital her daughter and her two eldest granddaughters went with her: 'I don't know who was more nervous, them or me. We sang all the way there in the taxi. I think the driver must have thought we were mad. The grandchildren are in their twenties, but were like two naughty little schoolgirls really. I think they were so scared . . . and then the nurse suggested that perhaps we would like to go and have a meal downstairs, which settled them down.'

Before the op, Sheila showered, put on her gown, and was given a pre-med sedative pill. She didn't remember any more after that until she woke up back on the ward. 'All I could think of was "I'm alive" and apparently I had a big grin on my face!' Her daughter came to see her on the third day and Sheila was reassured by her greeting: 'It was so nice 'cos she said, "Oh Mum, you do look well!" . . . By this time I felt so awake because before I had the op I was so tired.'

After the bypass, Sheila's recovery went quite smoothly, apart from suffering from vivid nightmares, and becoming a bit anxious and panicky at night when she first got back home: 'I found I had to leave the bedroom door open and the hall light on . . . even when one of the children was here.' But this phase didn't last long. As far as medication was concerned, she was kept on the same dosage of simvastatin (her cholesterol was now around 4.4 mmol/L). She also continued to take 75 mg aspirin, but the doctors felt that they could now control her blood pressure with a reduced dose of the ACE inhibitor lisinopril, and they were able to cut out the beta blocker – atenolol – altogether. Her blood pressure was now well controlled, with readings around 120/70 mm Hg, on just one 10 mg tablet of lisinopril a day rather than the 40 mg dose she needed before the bypass.

Sheila sums up her heart bypass experiences like this: 'The op's a definite plus . . . I didn't realize till after I'd had the op how ill I must have been . . . I had a cold the other weekend, and I thought, "What are you making a fuss about?" Because before . . . you still struggled and did things, and you could have dropped down dead. I'd say now, "Go and have it. You're going to be afraid. Yes, it is scary, but you come through the other side and you feel great. You really do!" I'm very pleased with myself!'

15
How bypass surgery affects the family

Coming to terms with the need for bypass surgery is not an isolated process. Most of those who are having bypass ops have a group of people surrounding them – partner, children (and grandchildren), parents, siblings and extended family. Or sometimes good friends rather than family may be the primary support. All of these people are influential in your life and they will also be influenced by you; and the way you interact will form an integral part of the rehabilitation process.

Family adjustment

Family adjustments need to be made, just as the person with the cardiac problems has had to adjust. Friends and family respond in their own individual ways, but reactions will generally be consistent, progressing through initial shock and disbelief, to grief, acceptance, adaptation and, finally, 'moving on' (see Chapter 6).

Sometimes the impact of a person's bypass operation on members of the family can be quite dramatic, affecting physical as well as psychological health. Robert (whose case is presented in Chapter 10) describes how his wife was affected: 'It's my wife I'm concerned about. She's wrecked. She's lost a lot of weight through all the worry of it all.' The physical and emotional demands on her had been great, but she was the person who had been most influential in keeping Robert in a positive frame of mind before the op, and helping him to make a speedy recovery afterwards.

Stephen (see Chapter 5) also owed a great deal to his wife, Deborah, who kept him buoyant before his op. She was pleased that Stephen was going to have the op, but it was still a big shock for the family: 'There was some relief but there was also a lot of fear 'cos you always think the worst. No matter what operation you have, you always tend to look on the black side in case something happens. With some operations, like the gall bladder removal, you can do without the bit they've taken out. But the heart, well, that's a bit special, isn't it? You're sort of preparing yourself, if you know what I mean.' Stephen takes up the story of the family's role after his bypass: 'I went in on Sunday night and came back the next Sunday.

The family were a terrific support. My wife came in every day – and the children. My brother drove us back home.'

The changes that take place within the dynamics of family life can have both positive and negative effects. In situations like Stephen's, it can have the effect of bringing the family closer together, but the stresses involved in having a family member in hospital can also bring increased tensions. Sheila (see Chapter 14) describes one episode that had a strong (though temporary) negative effect on the relationships between her children.

One of her daughters received news from the hospital that her mother's bypass had been successfully completed – but she failed to relay this to her other daughter: 'They had a flaming row and my son had to be the go-between!' All sorts of deep-seated sibling rivalries and other hidden family tensions can come to the fore in times of crisis. But the need to focus on the person who is undergoing treatment, rather than on their own relatively petty squabbles, can also help to strengthen family bonds. As Sheila says: 'Having to focus on my bypass probably brought the family closer together.'

Sometimes the illness of one partner can force a temporary change in roles between the partners. So the husband who had previously been the main bread-winner, and the person who always did DIY jobs and mowed the lawn, might be forced to stand aside for a while and watch while his wife performs some or all of these tasks. This may have the negative effect of making the wife feel overworked and stressed, while the husband stands on the sidelines criticizing his wife's efforts, like a disgruntled footballer recently dropped from the team, feeling humiliated that he's not able to play the role he considers that only *he* can play.

But there may be some positive outcomes too. The wife might find, for example, that she actually enjoys being outside mowing the lawn, while the husband's extra, 'enforced' spare time has given him the opportunity to re-kindle his interest in neglected pursuits, as with Peter (see Chapters 1 and 8) who 'got a bit more into reading, and took up fishing again'. By making an effort to seek out the positive advantages, it's often possible to turn a potential negative into a positive.

Communication

Talking through issues together regularly (as a couple, or with the children or the wider family) can expel myths, assumptions and negative beliefs that easily develop when individuals in the family are trying not to 'bother' each other with their worries. Although

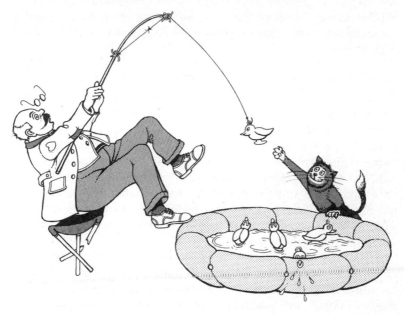

... and took up fishing again

keeping worries to ourselves is a common reaction when wanting to protect our family, it can also lead to underlying tensions that may spill out into arguments and squabbles.

Individuals within the family will tend to make assumptions about what they imagine others are thinking and feeling; but since it's impossible to read each other's minds, this leads to inaccurate perceptions, and sometimes a build-up of unspoken anger and resentment. Some of your reactions will have been a shock to you, and similarly your family's reactions may not be as you expect. Discussing issues more openly is a good way of avoiding this unhealthy build-up of negative emotion, or at least allowing the boil to be lanced!

Another common communication problem can arise when relatives don't listen to the wishes of the 'patient', but try to take over control themselves. They may want to 'wrap the patient up in cotton wool' because they are worried about them overdoing things. However, the 'patient' may feel quite happy getting on with new tasks and developing alternative roles while recovering at home. The failure to listen can lead to tension – something that can be diffused by allowing the person recovering from the bypass to express his or

111

her own views, and by discussing concerns openly. Disagreements will sometimes develop, but you can reduce them by adopting a communication style that is open-minded, supportive and 'listening' within the whole family.

Social support as an aid to recovery

Social support is one of the most well-recognized aids to the physical and emotional recovery from heart problems. Often it's just having a partner or close friend around that makes the biggest difference, as Robert explains: 'My wife's been a terrific support all through. She has taken a lot of the stress off me. Some of the phone-calls you need to make to sort out details about medicines and travel, for example, she's sorted all that out for me. That helps enormously.' Similarly, Peter says of his wife that 'she looks after me very well . . . When people say I'm looking well, I point to my wife and say "Well, there's my nurse"!'

All of us need support to cope with difficult events and circumstances in life and we need to think about the way in which we utilize it. Sometimes it can be useful to break down potential help into 'emotional' and 'practical' support – thinking about the people in our lives who are the good listeners, and those who can help with practical matters (e.g. DIY). It's also helpful to give people guidance about how they can best help you, providing them with useful feedback about how you view their role in your recovery. It will also help to diffuse any difficulties arising from family members trying to take on competing roles, which may be unhelpful or cause difficulties.

Sheila found that her children sometimes seemed to compete to look after her, although usually they took it in turns. Occasionally, though, one of them would object to doing something: 'My son came round to help me and he absolutely refused to help me have a bath. He said, "I'm not looking at you and your wrinkly bits, Mother." So his wife had to come round. But he was very good. He was like a sergeant-major. "Right, go and do a walk now, Mother . . . Do this . . . Go and have your rest . . ." I'm going to write a book one day about my experiences of my children when they looked after me.'

She also gained a lot of support from a lady she was in hospital with. 'We write to each other and she rings me up and I ring her up.' While recuperating, they compared experiences with one another, discussed progress, and shared problems in a mutually supportive manner.

Support for spouse/partner/main carer

Partners/spouses/main carers who are helping to look after the person with cardiac problems need their own separate support. Another family member, or a good friend or work colleague that you can trust, may fulfil this role. It is also important for the carer to be able to step away from the situation sometimes, to take both a physical and mental break away from the constant stresses and strains of caring. Space and time away allows a wider perspective through which it is easier 'to see the wood for the trees', and this will usually help to provide a smoother pathway through any difficulties.

Sometimes, the former 'patient' may find a way of repaying all the care he or she has received from relatives. We saw, for example, how Robert's wife lost a lot of weight worrying about his bypass, and how this concerned him at the time. He was pleased later on, however, when he was able to do something in return for all her support: 'She's now got to go into hospital for a small gynaecological op, and I've got to take on the supportive role. It'll probably be good for me, because you can get a bit self-obsessed. She put her op off until 12 weeks after I'd had mine. But it's my turn to give her the support she needs. Hope I'm as good as she was!'

If you can find your own effective ways of managing your physical health, and of coping with stressful situations along the lines discussed in the last few chapters, you will be well on your way to establishing a new healthy, high-quality post-bypass life.

16
Getting back to normal and maintaining a good quality of life

One query often raised by people who have had bypass operations is whether they'll ever 'get back to normal' and feel their 'old selves' again. They worry that they do not 'recognize' parts of themselves after undergoing bypass surgery. These 'unrecognizable selves' are often aspects of their personalities that came to the fore during the stresses of their surgery and rehab – some laudable and some less so! It is not surprising that those at the post-bypass stage should feel like this – going through an experience like a bypass operation is going to have effects that are both physical and psychological. But even if you have changed, this does not mean that you are not 'you'. Although you've found out new things about yourself and your family and friends, and have changed some areas of your lifestyle and ways of working, you're still 'you' – a different 'you' maybe, and possibly an improved 'you'!

Elements of your identity (who you are, what is important to you, what your values and principles are) may also have 'got lost' during your worrying 'bypass' journey. The rehabilitation period offers a useful time in which to reconsider these elements and to think about their importance in your life. You may also develop new aspirations that are fresh and challenging, and bring an energizing enthusiasm to your post-bypass life.

Peter (Chapters 1 and 8) describes a good example of someone who 'took off' after his bypass: 'He was older than me but he seemed to have loads of energy after his operation. He had a new lease of life and he took up fell walking . . . As a jazz musician he also went all over the place on gigs.'

Another key question is 'When can I get back to work?' Unfortunately, there are as many answers to this question as there are individuals who have undergone bypass operations! It depends entirely on the speed of recovery and the type of work involved. Someone working in an office performing light duties might expect to return sooner than someone working in a job involving heavy manual labour. But your doctor is unlikely to recommend that you return to work earlier than six weeks post-op, and for most people it's likely to be within eight to twelve weeks. As far as general fitness to return to work is concerned, your rehab staff will be able to offer you helpful advice.

For some people, experiencing life-threatening symptoms and undergoing surgery acts as a prompt for them to re-evaluate their lives. Those approaching retirement age, for example, may sometimes choose not to go back to work even though they are physically and mentally capable of doing so. Instead they might decide that the hiatus in their lives caused by their cardiac problems has offered them an opportunity to bring forward their retirement and to replace their daily work activities with other tasks and roles; for example, doing voluntary work, taking on new leisure activities or travelling. Other people, in contrast, will be very keen to return to work to give themselves a benchmark by which to assess their fitness level after the op, to have a part of their identity back again, and to earn a salary sufficient to maintain their usual standard of living.

Remember to pace your return just as you paced other activities during your rehab. For example, it's worth starting back at work on a part-time basis for a few weeks where this is feasible to allow you to ease your way back into your work routine. If you choose not to return, or were retired at the time of surgery, then it's important to make sure that your routine is structured and varied and contains the necessary elements for a fulfilling and rewarding quality of life. If you are choosing to bring forward your retirement, remember that this will also bring you face to face with issues associated with ageing and lifestyle change that you may not have considered before. Giving yourself time and space to adapt to, and prepare for, these new changes is an important part of your longer-term rehabilitation.

The concept 'quality of life' relates to your physical, emotional, social, financial and work-related well-being, each of which can impact on your general state of health; so it's important to consider all these elements in your efforts to maximize the positive outcomes of your bypass experience. You may find the idea that your physical *ill health* can have a *positive* spin-off a bit odd or ridiculous at first, but there will usually be some clear positive outcomes from your bypass experiences. Some people, like Sheila (page 45), will feel very strongly that the bypass has given them a 'second chance' and helped them to begin to value certain aspects of their lives that they had taken for granted, or ignored beforehand. They will often discover, for example, just how much love their families and friends have for them, and how much they love and value them in return. They may also thank the bypass experience for helping them to stop smoking and to start their new post-bypass life as a non-smoker –

115

without a morning cough, able to breathe more easily, and with their sense of taste restored so that they can fully enjoy the experience of eating the range of healthy foods on offer!

Emphasizing such positive elements of the 'bypass experience', and considering the things you have learned about yourself during this period, will provide valuable insights that you can build into your new life. They will also help you to feel comfortable about retaining your bypass experiences as memories that are not all bad.

After all the stress and strains of your bypass and rehabilitation, it's now *your* time to set off, like Peter's jazz musician friend, on your own 'special gigs'! The bypass has given you a second chance and the opportunities are there for you to take. Reflecting on, and learning about, how you coped with specific situations and problems during the bypass period will help you to cope with anything life can throw at you in the future. It's possible to enjoy an excellent quality of life after a bypass, and we hope that this book will help in your quest to achieve this.

Like the town dwellers who benefit so greatly from a new bypass relief road, which was the analogy used at the beginning of this book, we hope you will benefit from, and take pleasure in, the life-enhancing changes that your heart bypass can bring and the new horizons it can allow you to explore.

Enjoy your 'new gigs'!

Glossary

ACE inhibitors Class of drug that treats hypertension (high blood pressure) by inhibiting an Angiotensin Converting Enzyme. They help to reduce the constriction of the arteries and so reduce blood pressure.

Angina Cramp-like pain in the chest that comes on with exertion or overexcitement, caused by a restriction in blood flow to the heart.

Angiogram (coronary catheterization) Type of X-ray test in which a catheter (a small tube) is inserted in a vein or artery and fed through to the heart. Then a dye (visible on X-rays) is injected. The X-ray pictures indicating the state of the coronary arteries are shown on a video screen during the procedure.

Antioxidants A group of nutrients found in lots of fruit and vegetables, nuts, wine, grape juice and tea. They help to counteract the oxidization of substances such as cholesterol, which is less likely then to stick to the artery walls. They also counteract 'free radicals' which are implicated in other diseases such as cancer.

Anti-platelets Drugs, like aspirin, used to prevent the formation of clots in the blood vessels.

ARBs *(Angiotensin II Receptor Blockers; also called Angiotensin II Antagonists)* Class of drug similar to ACE inhibitors for treating hypertension.

Arrhythmias Abnormal heart rhythms. One of the most common is atrial fibrillation.

Atheromas Crusty deposits (plaques), mainly comprised of cholesterol, which clog up the arteries.

Atherosclerosis Condition in which the arteries become furred up and narrowed, with the build-up of atheroma plaques (see above). This process leads to heart disease.

Atrial fibrillation Abnormally fast and irregular heart rhythm in which upper chambers of the heart (the atria) start to 'quiver' (fibrillate).

Beta blockers Class of drug used to control blood pressure and/or angina by blocking some of the effects of adrenaline in our bodies.

Blood pressure Pressure of the blood against the artery walls.

Persistently high blood pressure (hypertension) is a risk factor for heart disease and stroke.

BMI Body Mass Index; formula used to identify a healthy weight/ height ratio.

CABG (Coronary Artery Bypass Grafting) Heart bypass operation in which the diseased sections of coronary arteries are replaced with healthy grafts taken from blood vessels in other parts of the body (e.g. leg, arm or the internal mammary artery).

Calcium antagonists Class of drugs for treating hypertension and/ or angina by reducing the amount of calcium available and thus helping to relax the blood vessels and reduce the heart's workload.

Cardiovascular disease (CVD) Disease of the cardiovascular system, including coronary heart disease and stroke.

Cardiovascular system The heart and its related blood vessels.

Cholesterol One of the fatty substances (lipoproteins or lipids) carried around in the blood. Mostly made in the liver from the fats we eat, especially saturated fat. It is essential to the healthy functioning of our bodies. There are two types: LDL (low density lipoprotein) and HDL (high density lipoprotein). Too much of the 'bad' LDL cholesterol tends to clog up the arteries, whereas the 'good' HDL cholesterol 'mops up' surplus cholesterol and helps to keep the arteries clear.

Coronary angioplasty Procedure for dilating a narrowed coronary artery. A catheter is inserted, as with the angiogram procedure, and a tiny balloon inflated at the point of constriction in the artery, and then withdrawn. *See also* Stent.

Coronary heart disease (CHD) Disease in which coronary arteries become clogged up, largely as a result of the build-up of atheromas.

Coronary thrombosis Blood clot blocking a coronary artery.

Diabetes Disease in which the body's ability to convert sugar from the foods we eat into energy (i.e. glucose metabolism) does not work efficiently.

Diuretics Category of drugs used to control blood pressure by increasing the amount of salt and water excreted in our urine, so reducing the volume of blood, and hence blood pressure.

ECG (Electrocardiogram) A test to check the rhythm and electrical activity of your heart. When this is carried out during exercise, this is called an exercise or stress ECG.

Echocardiography Examination of the heart by use of ultrasound scans.

Endarterectomy Scraping out plaque from an artery; often carried out on the carotid artery which feeds blood to the brain, when it is called carotid endarterectomy.

Familial hypercholesterolaemia (FH) Inherited genetic disorder in which levels of cholesterol are excessively high.

Glycaemic Index (GI) Measure applied to foods indicating effects on blood glucose levels. Foods with a *low* GI are an essential part of a heart-healthy diet.

HITS (High Intensity Transient Signals) Signals from a special ultrasound scanner (a Doppler machine) tracing the movement of plaque particles during a bypass operation.

Hypertension High blood pressure, as opposed to hypotension (low blood pressure).

MIDCAB (Minimally Invasive Direct Coronary Artery Bypass) Less 'invasive' procedure than the CABG since it is performed without a heart-lung bypass machine and without opening the breast bone. A small incision is made above the coronary artery and one of the internal mammary arteries is normally used to replace the diseased section.

Myocardial infarction (MI) Used to describe a heart attack – damage ('infarction') is caused to part of the muscular wall of the heart (the 'myocardium') because of a lack of blood supply resulting from a clot in a coronary artery.

OPCAB (Off-Pump Coronary Artery Bypass surgery) Like MIDCAB, a less invasive procedure than CABG that involves the use of special techniques that will keep part of the heart still without having to stop it completely. The heart-lung bypass machine is not usually required, but the breast bone still has to be opened.

Statins Collective name for a group of drugs used to lower cholesterol.

Stent Tiny tube made of stainless steel mesh, used to hold open narrowed coronary arteries and inserted as part of a procedure known as coronary angioplasty with stent.

Further reading and websites

A range of useful leaflets from the British Heart Foundation in their Heart Information Series is obtainable from the Foundation at 14 Fitzhardinge Street, London W1H 6DH or via their website (see below).

Further reading

Cheung, Theresa, *The Glycaemic Factor*. Sheldon Press, 2006.
Hartley, Mary, *Stress at Work*. Sheldon, 2003.
Povey, Robert, *How to Keep Your Cholesterol in Check* (3rd edn). Sheldon Press, 2006.
Povey, Robert, Morrell, Jacqui, and Povey, Rachel, *Eating for a Healthy Heart*. Sheldon Press, 2005.
Tubbs, Irene, *The Heart Recovery Book*. Sheldon Press, 2006.

Websites

ASH (Action on Smoking and Health): www.ash.org.uk

British Cardiac Patients' Association: www.bcpa.co.uk

British Heart Foundation: www.bhf.org.uk

Diabetes UK: www.diabetes.org.uk

Glycaemic Index: www.glycemicindex.com (information on index values)

H·E·A·R·T UK: www.heartuk.org.uk

Quit (smoking): www.quit.org.uk

Relaxation tape/CD: www.your-wellbeing.net/frames.html

Stroke Association: www.stroke.org.uk

Index